DATE DUE

~~OC 10 '97~~			
~~AP 2 '98~~			
~~AP 23 '01~~			
~~OC 10 01~~			
~~AP 2 '03~~			
~~JE 11 '03~~			
~~MY 12 '04~~			

DEMCO 38-296

The War Against Hepatitis B

The War Against Hepatitis B

A History of the International Task Force on Hepatitis B Immunization

William Muraskin

University of Pennsylvania Press

Philadelphia

cation Data

of the International Task
illiam Muraskin.

1d index.

1. International Task Force on Hepatitis B Immunization—History.
2. Hepatitis B—Vaccination—History.   3. International Task Force
on Hepatitis B Immunization.   I. Title.
   [DNLM: 1. Hepatitis B—history.   2. Hepatitis B—prevention &
control.   3. Hepatitis B Vaccines—history.   4. International
Cooperation.   WC 536 M972w   1995]
RA644.H4M87   1995
614.5′9362—dc20
DNLM/DLC
for Library of Congress   94-43276
                                                                CIP

Contents

Acknowledgments

I would like to thank the Research Foundation of the City University of New York for funding all the travel this project entailed. I especially want to thank Miriam Korman, who was my guardian angel at the Foundation. She lent a helping hand when I needed it the most.

I also want to thank Scott Halstead of the Rockefeller Foundation. His help and the generosity of the Rockefeller Foundation brought this book to fruition.

I am especially indebted to my editors Patricia Smith and Mindy Brown, who have gone out of their way to be supportive in all aspects of this endeavor, and whose help has been invaluable.

I am very grateful to the subjects of this book: Alfred Prince, James Maynard, Richard Mahoney, and Ian Gust, and all the other people associated with the International Task Force on Hepatitis B Immunization. They were not only extremely generous with their time, but also remarkably candid and open in sharing their views with me. I was deeply impressed by their willingness to allow an outsider free access to their files and papers. They took the position "paint us, warts and all," a risk-taking attitude as admirable as it is unusual. I especially want to thank Carol Jackson of the Program for Appropriate Technology in Health, whose help went beyond the call of duty.

I also appreciate the support that my colleagues at the Department of Urban Studies, Queens College, have shown me over the years, especially Steven Steinberg and the late Matthew Edel.

Lastly, I want to thank my wife, Merry, and my son, Michael, who put up with my constant travels—and did not protest when I did not ask them to come along!

Introduction

The AIDS epidemic has forced upon Americans the realization that the Age of Infectious Diseases is not a thing of the past—that the much-heralded miracles of twentieth-century medicine have not banished once and for all the plagues that periodically scourge mankind.[1] More than ten years before the appearance of AIDS, however, scientists—though not the general public—had already become aware of another viral pandemic that afflicted billions of people throughout the world and was responsible for massive death and morbidity. That disease, hepatitis B, also possessed a human reservoir—between two and three hundred million people—of infectious asymptomatic chronic carriers. Even worse, chronic carriership of the virus was highly associated with the later development of both cirrhosis and cancer of the liver. Indeed, the hepatitis B virus was found to be "the cause of up to 80% of all cases of hepatocellular carcinoma worldwide, second only to tobacco among known human carcinogens,"[2] and in countries without a high incidence of alcoholism, it was the primary cause of cirrhosis of the liver.

Hepatitis B virus infection can give rise to a wide variety of different outcomes. Its severity can range from inapparent cases no more severe than a mild flu to fulminating cases in which death occurs in a matter of days. In a significant number of cases "onset is . . . insidious with anorexia, vague abdominal discomfort, nausea and vomiting . . . often progressing to jaundice."[3] Hospitalization is often required in severe cases. Those infected with hepatitis can recover without even knowing they had been ill, or they can experience what feels like endless periods of lethargy and fatigue while recuperating. In more severe situations it can give rise to chronic hepatitis and years of disability during which the quality of life is totally undermined. If the individual becomes a chronic carrier of the virus he or she may lack noticeable symptoms for years and then experience increasing liver dysfunction, ultimately leading to cirrhosis or cancer (or both) and death. The younger a person is when infected by the hepatitis B virus, the higher the chances that he or she will become a chronic carrier. Asymptomatic cases are more likely to lead to carriership than clinically apparent ones. The severity of the clinical illness is greater when the infection is contracted by adults than by children. However, while children are more likely to remain asymptomatic, they are also more vulnerable to chronic carriership and the diseases to which it ultimately gives rise.[4] In the developing world, infection most often occurs during infancy and childhood; in the West infection most often is contracted during adulthood.

Cancer of the liver is the most devastating legacy hepatitis B imparts to its victims. Hepatocellular carcinoma is the leading cause of cancer deaths in the developing world. It strikes individuals, disproportionately men, in their most productive middle years, when the economic effect on their families and the larger economy is most destructive. While photojournalists' images of dying children are far more heart-rending to Westerners than pictures showing the demise of middle-aged men and women, the effect of adults' premature deaths is far more injurious to the social order. Couples can and do rapidly replace their young children, but children cannot readily replace their parents, or society its most economically productive members.

The existence of a worldwide pandemic can escape medical detection and public alarm when the scientific tools for its elucidation are lacking, or its natural signs are obscure or separated in time by decades. Such was the case with hepatitis B. Most infection in the developing world was "vertical," from mother to infant, or "horizontal," from person to person (usually a child), with nearly all cases of childhood infection being asymptomatic. When clinical cases did appear, they were difficult to distinguish from other diseases, especially hepatitis A—a less dangerous disease caused by a totally different virus but producing identical short-term symptoms. Its link to cancer and cirrhosis of the liver, sequelae that take thirty or forty years to appear after initial infection, was entirely hidden. Thus, it was for thousands of years a "silent" epidemic, whose dimensions and severity went unsuspected.

The most important research on hepatitis in the post–World War II period was done by Dr. Saul Krugman of New York University.[5] He became involved with hepatitis at Willowbrook, a residential institution for the mentally retarded in New York City. Krugman was called in to investigate what was believed to be a severe hepatitis A problem in the mid-1950s. Over time he demonstrated that the inmates of Willowbrook suffered from both hepatitis A and B, and he was able to confirm, in a way not done before, both the existence of two separate diseases and their contrasting characteristics. Among the things he demonstrated was that both diseases were infectious and thus that hepatitis B was not a purely iatrogenic illness but a contagious one that could be spread from person to person. In the late 1960s Krugman, in the final stages of his work, produced a proto-vaccine against hepatitis B by boiling contaminated human serum. He discovered that heating the liquid could kill the virus without adversely affecting its ability to provoke a protective antibody response. Most observers credit Krugman as the "father" of the hepatitis B vaccines that were developed after his pioneering work.[6]

The actual discovery of a blood test for the hepatitis B virus or, more accurately, the surface component of the virus was made accidentally by a geneticist, Dr. Baruch Blumberg. Blumberg was investigating possible genetic differences between ethnic and racial groups in their susceptibility to infectious diseases. As part of his work in the 1960s he encountered an unknown antigen in the blood of an Australian Aborigine, which he called the "Australian antigen." For a few years it was unclear what the antigen signified. Blumberg generated a number of theories consistent with his genetic interests, chief of which was that the antigen was a genetic human serum protein that made those who possessed it susceptible to a number of different diseases. Blumberg in 1966 collaborated with the virologist Alfred Prince of the New York Blood Center (NYBC), who had a long-term interest in transfusion hepatitis and suspected that the "Australian antigen" had a relationship to the hepatitis B virus. Ultimately, in the late 1960s a series of experiments established that a marker for the hepatitis B virus had indeed been discovered, which in turn meant that a blood test for the disease could be developed.

The newfound capability for readily identifying a marker for hepatitis B had a revolutionary impact on medical science. From that knowledge came in rapid succession (1) a test to protect the blood supply from "transfusion" hepatitis; (2) a tool for the full-scale investigation of the epidemiology and modes of transmission of the disease; and (3) the development of a safe and effective vaccine.

The epidemiological work carried out in the years after the hepatitis B virus blood test was developed revealed that the disease could be spread in a number of different ways, including from mother to child (perinatally), by sexual contact, through blood transfusions, and by intravenous drug use. In the 1980s, when the AIDS epidemic was first discovered, the similarity of transmission routes between the unidentified agent and the hepatitis B virus helped generate the hypothesis that there was a new viral agent spreading in the population. It also led to a quick formulation of "safe sex" guidelines for AIDS based upon the known ways of preventing hepatitis B transmission.

While discovery of the similarities between the transmission routes of hepatitis B and AIDS was vital in the early fight against human immunodeficiency virus (HIV) infection, there were significant differences as well. Hepatitis B is considerably more infectious than AIDS and can be spread in ways that AIDS cannot. Most importantly, hepatitis B can be spread by casual contact. In fact, most transmission of the disease in Africa, and even in Asia, is horizontal, from child to child. Children who play in unsanitary conditions with open sores or skin conditions or who come into close contact through cuts and skin breaks during play or fighting can and do spread the disease.

In addition, the hepatitis B virus is exceptionally hearty. It can maintain its infectiousness on environmental surfaces for months. It can be spread through the sharing of contaminated objects, such as towels, razors, chewing gum, hard candy, and fruit. It can be picked up from tattooing needles, ear-piercing instruments, blood-contaminated briar bushes, or key-punched computer cards. It can be spread by saliva as well as by sperm and vaginal fluids. Even minor breaks in the skin, such as those caused by hangnails, are sufficient to allow infection. Epidemiologists were appalled by the multitude of unexpected ways in which the disease could be passed from one person to another.

Researchers in the early 1970s discovered that the disease was ubiquitous in Asia and sub-Saharan Africa. In many countries 100 percent of the population would be infected at one point or another with hepatitis B. In some countries as much as 15 to 20 percent of the population would become chronic carriers of the disease, and it was estimated that one to two million people died each year from the chronic diseases that ultimately resulted.

In the West, hepatitis B was a far less common disease than in the developing world. Nevertheless, in the United States, for example, there were 200,000 to 300,000 cases of hepatitis B per year during the 1980s, and a carrier reservoir of approximately one million people. In the developed world, the disease was not normally contracted in childhood or infancy but rather during young adulthood. Most infection was contracted through sex (heterosexual or homosexual) or by intravenous drug use. However, there were literally dozens of non-sexually active or non-drug-using high-risk groups, from Down's syndrome children to morticians, from Eskimos to overseas armed forces personnel, from poor blacks to Chinese-Americans. One of the key high-risk groups included health care workers, especially those exposed to blood (e.g., surgeons, dentists, laboratory technicians, emergency room nurses, and pathologists). The number of occupations outside the field of health care that also had (an unnoticed) risk of blood exposure was surprisingly large and included police officers, fire fighters, sanitation workers, and hospital laundry employees.

The number of transmission routes, the stability of the virus outside the body, and the large numbers of at-risk groups initially raised great fear among medical researchers about the ability to contain the spread of the disease within the United States. They were especially worried about the dangers of health care workers spreading the disease to uninfected patients. This anxiety was magnified by the existence of the asymptomatic carrier state. There was very real fear in medical circles that if the general public became aware of the hepatitis B epidemic, massive discrimination against, and stigmatization of, carriers might result. They were especially concerned about the danger of the creation of a new "leper class" that would include even the most prestigious health care professionals.

The response of the American health care community to the hepatitis B situation was to try to "contain" knowledge of the danger to itself and to other groups at high risk of carriership. The medical authorities took the position that until clear and unequivocal evidence showed that carriers posed a danger to the public health, it should be assumed that they did not, and that careful hygiene and education would protect against transmission. They recommended little or no restrictions on the normal lives and occupations of carriers. (This approach has remained to this day practically free from criticism except in my own writings on hepatitis B, where I have argued that its "see no evil, speak no evil" attitude has needlessly endangered the public's health.[7] Among other things, I have emphasized the conflict of interest inherent in having one of the high-risk groups for hepatitis B carriership—i.e., health professionals—determine policy for dealing with those chronically infected with the disease.)

The rapid development of a safe and effective vaccine by 1982 appeared to support the wisdom of the go-it-alone strategy, seemingly providing a solution to most aspects of the hepatitis B problem both in the West and in the developing world. Perhaps even more important, because of the role the hepatitis B virus plays in the origin of hepatocellular carcinoma, *the new vaccine constituted for all practical purposes the first effective anti-cancer vaccine ever developed.* It was one of the great triumphs of modern science that the time between the development of a test for the virus and production of a commercial vaccine was little more than a decade, and the hepatitis B vaccine proved to be one of the safest vaccines ever developed.

Unfortunately, the development of the vaccine did not lead to a major offensive against the worldwide hepatitis B pandemic. This great achievement of medicine and technology turned out to have little practical effect, though not because of any inherent weaknesses within the scientific enterprise. The epidemic continued unabated throughout the developing world. Indeed, even in the United States, the incidence of hepatitis B cases rose from 200,000 to 300,000 cases a year in the period immediately following the licensing of the vaccine (in 1982). This escalation of the epidemic in America occurred despite the radical decrease in number of cases among homosexuals after their adoption of anti-AIDS "safe sex" practices. The decrease in number of cases among homosexuals was more than offset by the increase among heterosexuals with multiple partners, a population that then replaced homosexuals as the highest at-risk group. The vaccine was utilized by too few people, even among health care workers who, unfortunately, were practically the only people aware that there was both an epidemic and a preventative against it. Something had gone very wrong.

A number of problems existed that made a successful fight against hepatitis B impossible, not the least of which was the low profile (i.e., public obscurity) that the American medical authorities encouraged. The biggest obstacle, however, was the exorbitant price of the vaccine. The vaccine cost more than $100 for the required three shots. Such a price exceeded the yearly family income in many developing countries, let alone government budgets for health expenditure. Even in the United States this price put it outside the range of what most people would pay. The high cost of hepatitis B immunization not only made it impossible for individuals and governments to take advantage of the new scientific breakthrough, it also made it unaffordable for international agencies such as the World Health Organization (WHO), UNICEF (the United Nations Children's Fund), or the donor groups that funded their work.

The vaccine was priced exorbitantly because of the politics of commercial vaccine development. As already mentioned, a proto-vaccine was produced by Saul Krugman by simply boiling the blood of a known hepatitis B carrier. While Krugman decided not to work on perfecting his unexpected discovery, Baruch Blumberg proceeded to develop his own version of the vaccine and went on to patent it in 1969. Blumberg then waited for a pharmaceutical company to develop a commercial version. Merck and Company was attracted to the project, but Blumberg discovered that the drug manufacturer was not interested in the vaccine unless it could have exclusive patent rights. Because of the nature of Blumberg's funding from the National Institutes of Health (NIH), he was forbidden to give any company a monopoly over the vaccine. As a result Merck lost interest and withdrew—for five years. The Blumberg vaccine sat on the shelf, useless. (In the interim, NIH itself worked on a hepatitis B vaccine but could only license, not sell, it; it discovered that, like Merck, no drug company would get involved without a guarantee of exclusive rights over the patent.)

Finally, in the mid-1970s, a way around the government's restrictions on patent use was found. Merck was given exclusive rights over the vaccine in markets outside the United States. Only with that guarantee did the company proceed to invest in making a commercial hepatitis B vaccine. There were clearly many practical obstacles to overcome, and the work was carried out at a very high level under the formidable guidance of Maurice Hilleman at Merck. Nevertheless, the price Merck finally decided to charge came as shock to scientists in the field. No one knows how much Merck spent on developing the final product—those records are a business secret. Clearly, however, Merck did not have to spend large amounts of money on basic research, the groundbreaking work having been done by others using government funds. Many believed that the vaccine could be economically produced for as low as $1–2 a dose and still turn a profit. (Ultimately critics of the high-priced vaccine would discover that in sufficiently large quantities the cost per unit could fall to as low as ten cents a dose.)

The key problem for those concerned about the public health implications of the hepatitis B vaccine was that the American government would not manufacture such vaccines itself. It could directly develop them or help outside researchers work on them, but it would not allow itself to compete with the private sector. It is an example of what the historian Robert Lively has called "the American System"[8]: the government invests in research and development when entrepreneurs are hesitant because of the high risk or lack of quick payback, but withdraws in favor of the private sector when profits are obtainable; the government thus functions as an aid to business but not as a competitor. This system, in one form or another, has operated for more than 200 years and clearly has many virtues, but it does not guarantee low prices for the public nor equitable access for the poor.

During the 1970s and 1980s the U.S. government, as well as its public health service, was under severe financial pressure. Funds were being cut and money was lacking for research, prevention, and treatment of many diseases—even the most common and least costly to deal with. The swine flu immunization fiasco made matters considerably worse for researchers, especially those looking for funds to fight a "new" disease. Hepatitis B, for a variety of reasons, became increasingly labeled as a disease of "outsiders"—since the most prominent high-risk groups in America were homosexual and bisexual men and intravenous drug users—which made arguments for spending money on it potentially unpopular.

Many concerned public health experts found the hepatitis B situation in the United States extremely frustrating. Even more exasperating was the situation outside the country, where the high-priced vaccine was most desperately needed and most unaffordable.

The Purpose of This Book

Such was the situation when a group of scientists decided to take action into their own hands and find a way to make affordable mass immunization a reality in the developing world, where most cases of hepatitis B existed. This book is the story of that unusual group of socially conscious scientists and their organization, the International Task Force on Hepatitis B Immunization. It is the story of how a few strong-willed and determined individuals radically changed the lives of millions of people.

The following chapters attempt to accomplish a number of different tasks. An accurate record is presented of what will someday be seen as one of the great scientific achievements of the twentieth century—the practical implementation of a program to eradicate one of the world's most widespread viral diseases and, with it, the predominant cancer in the Third World. It also gives a detailed look at the extreme difficulties of working in the international arena where competing interests on local, national, and global levels continually interfere with the creation of effective programs. This book provides a unique "insider" look at the politics of world health because I was given unlimited access to the International Task Force's confidential files. It is very rare for a historian to have totally uncensored access to such delicate material from a key player on the international stage.

The book will show that the individuals who created the Task Force had long been dedicated to fighting the hepatitis pandemic or working to alleviate oppressive health problems in the developing world. The experience, knowledge, and scientific and political sophistication they had acquired over time made it possible for them to create a task force that was so potent that it could rearrange the priorities of the international health agenda.

The organization they created was able to take advantage of a limited window of opportunity that existed in the pharmaceutical industry as the result of the emergence of the newly industrialized countries on the Pacific Rim. The decision of Korean manufacturing companies to enter the international arena aggressively to compete with established Western and Japanese corporations provided the Task Force with the possibility of using that rivalry to lower the price of the vaccine radically—the sine qua non of any mass immunization campaign.

The Task Force was able to defend the scientific legitimacy of the new Asian "cheap" vaccines, while simultaneously working to convince Western manufacturers to accept low (unit) profits in a massive lower-class market rather than to seek high (unit) profits in a restricted elite market.

While striving to affect positively the policies adopted by vaccine suppliers, the Task Force also labored to educate and inspire the potential consumers of the vaccine—the governing elites of developing nations. They established elaborate model immunization projects in both Asia and Africa (Indonesia, Thailand, China, Kenya, and Cameroon). The models were designed to demonstrate that it was possible to reach and immunize an entire cohort of newborns during the first week of life, even in isolated rural areas; to find and solve the myriad of practical problems that large-scale immunization programs face under actual field conditions; to educate neighboring countries to the significance of hepatitis B; and to inspire them to initiate similar programs.

The Task Force championed a culturally sensitive approach to working with and motivating host governments. It emphasized the importance of obtaining detailed knowledge of the various political and social forces in each country so that supporters could be energized and opponents neutralized or won over. In some countries it acted primarily as a catalyst for existing forces that desired to combat the hepatitis B epidemic but were unable to initiate action without the aid of external pressure; in others it worked to bring such forces into existence.

While working on both the suppliers and potential users of hepatitis B vaccine, the Task Force also had to deal with the key international agencies (WHO and UNICEF) that are the vital intermediaries between the pharmaceutical companies and the developing world. Especially in its dealings with WHO, the Task Force had to tread a fine line between being an ally and a critic. WHO held the general mandate from the United Nations to deal with the world's health problems, of which hepatitis B was but one; yet, it lacked the resources or expertise to carry out such an all-encompassing obligation successfully. WHO clearly needed help, but the politics of international health made it difficult for it to accept aid without a significant loss of face. The International Task Force on Hepatitis B Immunization by its very existence implied a failure on the part of WHO. It was thus incumbent upon the new group to exercise exceptional tact when dealing with WHO so as not to alienate its leaders permanently.

While the following chapters will fill in the details of the Task Force's activities, this book will also try to answer the question of whether activist scientists and public health workers can do for other diseases what has been done for hepatitis B. I believe that the history of the Task Force will demonstrate that its work is repeatable in the future for other major diseases; thus, scientists acting in the political arena can positively affect policy decisions.

The Task Force members were driven by a powerful moral sense of urgency, fueled by the knowledge that 2,000 to 5,000 people die each day from cancer or cirrhosis of the liver because of a hepatitis B virus infection they contracted in childhood. Nevertheless, their success could only come from their ability to combine that potentially impractical fervor with a pragmatic willingness to work within the international system and play hard-headed institutional politics. The power to achieve universal hepatitis B vaccine immunization rested with WHO, the Expanded Programme on Immunization (EPI), UNICEF, dozens of Third World governments, and the cooperation of at least some commercial pharmaceutical companies. The Task Force often actively confronted those powerful international players and frequently pressured, embarrassed, and "forcefully" educated them. However, the Task Force lacked the power to bring about internal political change among the groups it dealt with. Rather, it had to work with the elites that were in place.

A Brief Look at the Context Within Which the Task Force Operated

The international structure for the large-scale delivery of vaccines to the developing world, upon which the Task Force wished to make its mark, was a highly divided and contentious one, whose shape had been formed only recently. The system developed in part out of the cooperative activities of WHO, UNICEF, and the Rockefeller Foundation in the 1950s. The three organizations decided to launch a coordinated campaign against yaws, a tropical disease that often afflicted children. It was a highly successful joint effort, which was followed by other campaigns against leprosy, trachoma, and tuberculosis.[9] The experiences gained from those activities provided support for the idea that international collaboration against infectious diseases could be successful.

In keeping with that hope, the World Health Assembly of WHO in 1955 declared a worldwide effort to eradicate malaria. The program, which promised to be one of the great achievements of mankind, ended in severe disappointment. The new program and its early successes led many countries to abandon traditional malaria control methods, replacing them with massive applications of DDT. The absence of continuous vigilance, combined with the demise of traditional control methods, the scattering of malaria experts, and the growth of DDT-resistant strains, produced a disastrous resurgence of the disease; in many places it became more severe than it had originally been.[10]

The failure at malaria eradication was interpreted as an object lesson in the dangers of conducting the "wrong type" of health program:

If single-focused—vertical—programs are not sustainable by virtue of being part of continuing primary health services all they achieve is a vacuum. . . . Even control of a disease, much less its eradication, needs eternal vigilance. . . . If . . . [the disease] doesn't vanish, . . . [people] become disillusioned and apathetic.[11]

Despite the depressing lessons of this first eradication campaign, and the wariness that resulted from it, WHO embarked on a second vertical campaign in 1959. The second international offensive was aimed at smallpox. In this case, the World Health Assembly acted more cautiously, taking no action until after smallpox had been successfully eradicated in Europe and North America, and there were encouraging results from efforts in the Philippines and both Central and South America. The ambitious program, however, was insufficiently supported, and it failed.[12]

If things had remained at this point there never would have been an international system geared to supplying the developing world with any vaccines, let alone hepatitis B. However, in the late 1960s a third attempt at a massive international intervention against an infectious disease was launched—once again against smallpox. That effort was a striking success.

The second smallpox eradication effort grew out of the activities of the U.S. Communicable Disease Center (CDC) [later the Centers for Disease Control] and the U.S. Agency for International Development (USAID). Both groups were frequently involved in helping the developing world combat infectious diseases. As a result of negotiations between the two agencies they became involved in fighting smallpox in West Africa. The resulting CDC-USAID effort helped create pressure to extend the fight from Africa into Asia.[13]

In 1967 the World Health Assembly again declared war against smallpox. The effort was headed by Donald Henderson, a member of the CDC and veteran of the West Africa program.[14] Despite the trauma of the malaria campaign, the smallpox effort was a classical "vertical" program—a single-focus project aimed at a disease, in which outsiders entered a country to help indigenous authorities in an intense but nonsustainable effort. Some in WHO had severe reservations about such programs on ideological grounds—preferring projects that built lasting health structures, whereas others at WHO "viewed the smallpox program negatively [simply] because it ran outside the regular WHO system."[15]

The smallpox program involved many different groups working together, but not always harmoniously. Many of the personnel for the WHO-sponsored program came from the CDC. The CDC people had an individualistic style that was often at odds with the rule-conscious, bureaucratic temperament of WHO workers. In Latin America the Pan-American Health Organization (PAHO) was active, and while it was technically the representative of WHO in the Americas, a significant amount of jealousy and rivalry still existed between the two organizations. There was also conflict between the CDC and USAID, with the former more action-oriented than the latter.[16]

The results of the campaign were many and far-reaching. Of greatest significance was that it proved effective international cooperation was possible on a grand scale, and that an infectious disease could be totally eradicated by design. It also "left [behind] an experienced group of health officials ready to continue programs against malaria, diarrhea, blindness, vaccine-preventable diseases, and other health programs."[17]

Many of the members of the WHO staff that served under Donald Henderson during the smallpox campaign commented that it was unfortunate that they had not been armed with other vaccines so that they could deliver them at the same time.[18] This sentiment was obviously shared by others, because in 1974 WHO established its EPI to encourage the developing world to vaccinate its children against six vaccine-preventable diseases: polio, diphtheria, pertussis, tetanus, tuberculosis, and measles. The head of the new program was Ralph Henderson, one of Donald Henderson's deputies during the smallpox program.[19]

EPI would form the backbone of the new international vaccine-delivery system. There has been controversy over the true nature of EPI, because it appears to be a typical "vertical" program (emphasizing the targeting of specific diseases) rather than a "horizontal" one that concentrates on the delivery of general primary health care or the fostering of across-the-board economic development. As we will see in a later chapter, the fight between "vertical" and "horizontal" approaches to health has been a long and bitter one that has divided the international health community. WHO has been generally hostile to vertical programs, in keeping with the lessons it learned from the anti-malaria campaign and the general philosophy of Halfdan Mahler, one of its most influential Directors-General.[20] Mahler was outspoken in his hostility to scientific "fixes" and eloquent in his support for primary health care and general economic development as the key to world health.

However, EPI has been a vertical program with a major difference. Establishment of a permanent vaccine delivery system in the nations of the developing world has been its dedicated goal. It has radically opposed one-shot campaigns that target an area and then pack up and leave when it is over. EPI has been willing to work only in areas with adequate health infrastructure already in place, or where the government is willing to establish such a structure, and has striven to be integrated into the primary health care system (horizontal programs) or to become the core around which such a system can be created. Sustainability has been its creed, and in that respect the ideological conflict between vertical and horizontal approaches has not been truly relevant to it. Because of its unique combination of qualities, Mahler was very supportive of both EPI and its leader, Ralph Henderson,[21] something that has not been appreciated by all observers.[22]

The WHO EPI under Henderson labored carefully and cautiously to encourage countries in the developing world to establish their own national EPIs. The international EPI did not have the resources or the mandate to create its own centralized system. Rather, its job was to persuade local elites of the need for vaccination, then to train cadres of workers (at the international, regional, and national levels) who could establish and maintain a vaccine delivery system. The Geneva-based EPI also worked to perfect the technology needed to deliver vaccines effectively (e.g., the hardware to maintain the cold chain that preserves vaccine efficacy) and to make that knowledge available to developing countries. The national EPIs would then establish effective delivery systems, starting in those areas where they could maintain the cold chain and slowly expand until they could successfully cover their entire countries. In the years after 1974 Henderson and his people (in Geneva and in the individual nations) methodically and carefully moved forward.

However, the growth of immunization rates in the developing world was very slow. Many observers became impatient with the limited progress made. As we will see in Chapter 2, Kenneth Warren of the Rockefeller Foundation argued as early as 1979 that the health community should concentrate more of its efforts on immunization in the fight to combat child mortality, since alternative policies were, tragically, less effective.

In 1982 UNICEF made a forceful entrance into the health field by declaring "the Children's Revolution" and proceeding to champion a series of health measures. It thus laid a claim to an area that up to then had been the preserve of WHO. This was a situation bound to cause conflict. As a result of conversations among James Grant, head of UNICEF, Kenneth Warren of Rockefeller, Robert McNamara (an ex-president of the World Bank), and Jonas Salk, an international conference was convened at Bellagio, Italy, in 1983, with the goal of championing the cause of immunization, influencing WHO's priorities, and forcefully accelerating the pace of EPI's growth by staging a series of dramatic national vaccination campaigns.[23]

Out of the Bellagio conference, and two subsequent conferences, came a new determination on the part of the international health community to promote aggressively mass immunization of the world's children against the six diseases that EPI had targeted. At that point UNICEF committed itself to helping raise the funds to purchase the vaccines—a vital goal if the percentage of immunized children was to be significantly raised. At the same time the United Nations Development Programme, UNICEF, and the Rockefeller Foundation formed a new organization, the Task Force for Child Survival, with the hope that they could coordinate their efforts and maintain the increased momentum. In all the new activities, the participants exerted considerable effort to make it possible for UNICEF and WHO to cooperate, despite their rivalry in matters of health and their differing attitudes toward vertical and horizontal programs (UNICEF favored the former and WHO the latter).

The result of all this activity was that the long-term utopian goal of immunizing all the world's children with the EPI's six universal vaccines started to look like a reality. However, the growing national EPI infrastructures suggested the possibility that new vaccines could be quickly added to the network as they were developed.[24]

This was the environment within which the International Task Force on Hepatitis B Immunization had to maneuver. WHO, EPI, and UNICEF were the key international players that had to be won over if universal hepatitis B vaccination were to become a reality. Since the various groups had conflicting attitudes and interests that had to be accommodated, the Task Force had to tread very carefully in dealing with them.

There were, in addition, other important players who also had to be carefully wooed, including the Task Force for Child Survival, the Rockefeller Foundation, USAID, Rotary International, and the foreign aid agencies of Canada, Australia, and Japan—to name just a few of the most prominent governmental donor groups. The following chapters attempt to illuminate how the Task Force could, against all odds, successfully champion its cause in this complex and contentious milieu.

A major insight into the Task Force's ability to work fruitfully, not only on the highest international level but also in specific countries in the Third World (Thailand, Indonesia, Kenya, and Cameroon), can be gleaned by noting the similar attributes possessed by the Task Force and the leaders of the smallpox eradication campaign. According to Jack Hopkins, one of the chroniclers of the latter program, the struggle proved winnable because its managers possessed flexibility, openness to feedback from the field, sensitivity to the culture and politics of the local country, an interest in educating the local population and encouraging local community participation, a concern for the need to assess and evaluate results continually, a compulsive concern for details, and an ability to combine idealism and realism.[25] As the following chapters will demonstrate, these attributes also perfectly describe the core qualities of the International Task Force on Hepatitis B Immunization as it worked in the developing world.

A Word About the Author and the Task Force

Before beginning, a comment about my own relationships to the International Task Force on Hepatitis B Immunization is necessary. This book focuses on real and perceived conflicts of interest that have affected international health policy, and I feel I must make clear my own relationship to my subjects.

I had been doing research on the hepatitis B epidemic in the United States for a number of years before I learned of the existence of the International Task Force. In fact, my first awareness of the organization came during an interview at WHO in Geneva, where it was mentioned in a throw-away comment, unexpectedly dropped into the conversation. Most of my writing up to that point had been highly critical of the way the hepatitis B epidemic had been handled in the United States. I kept wishing that someone would take an aggressive approach to the epidemic, in opposition to the cautious, self-protective way that seemed to dominate American policies.

Much of my enthusiasm for the Task Force derives from the contrast I found between the halting effort in the United States and the dynamic activity of the Task Force. However, despite starting out with a positive attitude toward the organization, I was determined to maintain complete freedom to evaluate the group's work. I wished to see proof that it lived up to its initial promise. I was especially anxious that I not lose my independence as the price of obtaining unrestricted access to their confidential records. As a result, we agreed that I would receive no financial or other support from the Task Force, other than the freedom to rummage through its files and pester its personnel with a deluge of questions. The only exception to this agreement was that the Task Force was kind enough to accept the charges for a multitude of long-distance phone calls from New York to Task Force-PATH headquarters in Seattle as I attempted to have further questions answered and facts updated. One of the things I admire about the Task Force's leadership is the great risk they were willing to take by having an outsider examine their records in the absence of any protection from what he might write about them.

Notes

1. Much of the Introduction is based on the following sources: William Muraskin, "The Silent Epidemic: The Social, Ethical, and Medical Problems Surrounding the Fight Against Hepatitis B," *Journal of Social History* 22 (1988): 277–298; idem, "Individual Rights Versus the Public Health: The Controversy over the Integration of Retarded Hepatitis B Carriers into the New York City Public School System," *Journal of the History of Medicine and Allied Sciences* 45 (1990):64–98; idem, "Individual Rights Versus the Public Health: The Problem of the Asian Hepatitis B Carriers in America," *Social Science and Medicine* 36 (1993):203–216; idem, "Hepatitis B as a Model (and Anti-Model) for AIDS," in *AIDS and Contemporary History,* edited by Virginia Berridge and Philip Strong (New York: Cambridge University Press, 1993), 108–132; and idem, "The Willowbrook Experiments Revisited: Saul Krugman and the Politics of Morality" (unpublished manuscript, available from the author). Other sources are noted when relevant.

2. Abram S. Benenson, ed., *Control of Communicable Diseases in Man* (Washington, D.C.: American Public Health Association, 1985), 171.

3. Benenson, *Control of Communicable Diseases,* 171.

4. Ibid.

5. Krugman's work built upon the research achievements of scientists during World War II. During the war many American servicemen were inoculated against yellow fever with a vaccine that contained human serum, and as an unexpected by-product of that vaccination thousands of them came down with hepatitis. For many years there had been evidence that a form of hepatitis existed that was transmitted by injections and transfusions rather than in the "natural" way. This suggested an iatrogenic disease caused by Western medical technology. It became important for the military to know the relationship between "serum" or "transfusion" hepatitis (ultimately called hepatitis B) and the more common "infectious" hepatitis (ultimately called hepatitis A).

The lack of a test for the causative agent for either disease (and it was not clear that they were truly separate diseases, as opposed to strains of the same disease) made the work quite difficult. Without an animal model, or an identified agent that could be cultured in the laboratory, investigators were forced to use human subjects in experiments designed to uncover the characteristics, modes of transmission, and relationship between the two hypothesized viruses. Subjects were exposed to contaminated material by a variety of routes—inoculation with blood, ingestion of fecal material, etc.—and the results were observed. Since investigators had no tests to prove definitively the presence of the different agents, they had to assume, sometimes incorrectly, that the material they used was contaminated with only one or the other virus. The result of painstaking detective work was the generation of a series of remarkably, though not totally, accurate hypotheses: there were two different viral agents, one passed primarily through the oral-fecal route and the other by blood transfer; infection with either strain provided immunity from re-infection by the same strain but not cross-immunity with the other one; and there was an asymptomatic carrier state for the blood-borne hepatitis (hepatitis B), though not for the oral-fecal type.

6. Krugman's experiments at Willowbrook became the center of a major controversy in the mid-1960s when charges were made that his work with the retarded was an example of unethical medical research. A consensus formed

among academics that the charges were true, and ever since his work on hepatitis has been used in textbooks on medical ethics as an example of abhorrent research. This negative interpretation of Krugman's work and character has always been rejected by the vast majority of those working in the infectious disease research community. They have continued for the last thirty years to lionize and honor him and his contributions to controlling childhood diseases. My own research on Willowbrook does not support the jaundiced evaluations of academic observers; rather it leads me to believe that Krugman was scapegoated in an almost biblical fashion by reformers who worked to replace the then-existing ethical system controlling medical research with a rival system. Krugman was caught in the middle of a "sea change" in values as reformers moved toward instituting a radically egalitarian, individual rights–dominated ethical code to replace the existing one, which was more hierarchial, utilitarian, and community obligation-oriented. See Muraskin, "The Willowbrook Experiments Revisited: Saul Krugman and the Politics of Morality."

7. One limited exception to this silence came from the New York City Health Department. For details see Muraskin, "Individual Rights Versus the Public Health: The Controversy over the Integration of Retarded Hepatitis B Carriers into the New York City Public School System."

8. Robert Lively, "The American System," *Business History Review* 29 (1955): 81–94.

9. See June Goodfield, *A Chance to Live: The Heroic Story of the Global Campaign to Immunize the World's Children* (New York: Macmillan, 1991), 27.

10. See *The Cambridge World History of Human Disease,* edited by Kenneth F. Kiple (Cambridge: Cambridge University Press, 1993), 861; and Goodfield, *A Chance to Live,* 28–29.

11. Goodfield, *A Chance to Live,* 29.

12. See Jack W. Hopkins, *The Eradication of Smallpox: Organizational Learning and Innovation in International Health* (Boulder, Colo.: Westview Press, 1989), 6–7.

13. Ibid., 8.

14. Goodfield, *A Chance to Live,* 24.

15. Hopkins, *Eradication of Smallpox,* 50.

16. Ibid., 50, 54, 56, 58.

17. Ibid., 49.

18. Goodfield, *A Chance to Live,* 24.

19. Ibid., 29.

20. For example, see Goodfield, *A Chance to Live,* passim.

21. John Clements of EPI said that Henderson came in with Mahler and a significant part of the EPI's vision came from Mahler. Mahler gave Henderson a great deal of freedom, "fully knowing what kind of man Henderson was" (interview with Clements, July 9, 1990). Also, James Maynard, ex-Chief of the Hepatitis Branch, CDC, and a leader of the International Task Force on Hepatitis B, said that anyone who says EPI was not fully supported by WHO is entirely mistaken (interview with Maynard, November 12, 1993).

22. Goodfield in her influential book *A Chance to Live* gives the impression that since WHO generally, and Mahler specifically, were so opposed to vertical programs, the EPI was less than enthusiastically supported (p. 33). In addition, her book severely distorts the role of the EPI. Despite writing about the campaign to immunize the world's children, she almost never refers to the EPI by name; she simply talks about "WHO." Unfortunately, since most of the book is

structured as a comparison between UNICEF's promotion of vertical programs and WHO's championship of horizontal programs, EPI's unique qualities are ignored. The reader is often left to wonder if the "WHO" in any given paragraph is the EPI or the anti-vertical parts of the WHO bureaucracy. Even more important, it is almost impossible to glean from Goodfield's account that UNICEF's chief contributions to immunizing the world's children (e.g., its commitment to financing large-scale purchases of vaccines for EPI, and the creation of high-profile, short-term campaigns designed to build popular and elite support for the national EPIs) depended upon the existence of the EPI for their success. UNICEF could neither supplant nor bypass the EPI structure or achieve any lasting improvement without it. EPI may have needed to be pushed and reinvigorated by outsiders to become truly effective, but it was still the core vehicle for immunization. This fact is obscured by Goodfield's treatment and mars her otherwise informative book. David Parker and Terrel Hill, of UNICEF, present a much more accurate perspective on the roles played by EPI and UNICEF in their paper "The Contribution of Immunization to Economic Development," presented at the Conference on Vaccines and Public Health, Bethesda, Maryland, November 5–6, 1992, sponsored by the National Institute of Allergy and Infectious Diseases.

23. Goodfield, *A Chance to Live,* 39. Also see Chapter 2 of this book for Warren's account of the origin of the Task Force for Child Survival, which differs in some particulars from Goodfield's.

24. Interview with Ralph Henderson, Assistant Director-General of WHO, ex-Director of EPI, July 10, 1990.

25. See Hopkins, *Eradication of Smallpox,* especially 125–134.

Chapter 1
The Formative Years

The International Task Force on Hepatitis B Immunization came into existence because of the determination, stubbornness, and idealism of four dynamic and strong-willed individuals. They became founders of this organization through a variety of separate though continually intersecting routes. The expert knowledge, political sophistication, and broad appreciation of Third World peoples that each acquired on his own would make it possible for them to create an organization capable of changing world health priorities.

The four men who founded the Task Force were Drs. Alfred Prince, James Maynard, Ian Gust, and Richard Mahoney. In the period before the Task Force's formation, each had attained significant success in furthering the cause of fighting hepatitis B or improving general health conditions in the developing world, but each was frustrated by the limited nature of his accomplishments. The combination of achievement and frustration would force each of them to search for a more effective means of influencing international health policy.

The best place to begin the story of the Task Force is not at its formal creation but in the years before the founders came together as a group. One of the striking aspects of their lives during that period was how often their paths crossed. Without a conscious plan, they forged personal and professional bonds, the true import of which would only appear at a later time.

The Task Force would ultimately crystallize around the person of Alfred Prince and his innovative vaccine technology. It is therefore logical to begin this study with an investigation of Prince and his attempts to combat the hepatitis B pandemic.

Alfred Prince

Alfred Prince, M.D., of the New York Blood Center (NYBC), the future Chairman of the Task Force, was an internationally renowned virologist who had sought out the causes of hepatitis since the late 1950s. He was one of the three key researchers (the other two being Drs. Saul Krugman and Baruch Blumberg) whose work made it possible to differentiate clearly between infectious hepatitis (hepatitis A) and serum hepatitis (hepatitis B), develop a diagnostic blood test for hepatitis B, and lay the groundwork for development of a vaccine. In 1966 Blumberg asked Prince to investigate a possible relationship between the "Australian antigen" and hepatitis. As a result of this research, Prince was the first person to become convinced that this antigen was intimately related to hepatitis as opposed to leukemia or some other disease, and that its chief significance lay in the field of virology rather than genetics, which was Blumberg's specialty. Blumberg and Prince's collaboration came to an acrimonious end when Prince insisted that they publish an article identifying the Australian antigen specifically with hepatitis. At that time Blumberg was unwilling to relinquish his hypothesis that the antigen was a genetically produced human protein that made the individual susceptible to leukemia, leprosy, hepatitis, and so forth.[1]

Though Prince was an indefatigable researcher, he avoided the isolation of the ivory tower scientist because of his fierce social beliefs. He had long maintained that the discoveries of the laboratory should benefit mankind, not simply boost careers, make profits, or produce monographs to grace the pages of scholarly publications. His social commitment had deep personal roots, going back to pre–World War II Germany where his father, in a manner not uncommon among middle-class Jews, combined the vocation of businessman with an allegiance to the principles of democratic socialism. Prince has spent most of his adult career at the non-profit NYBC, trying to live in harmony with many of those parental ideals.

Prince, along with both Blumberg and Krugman, was quick to realize the feasibility of creating a hepatitis B vaccine from infected plasma.[2] Blumberg acted first and patented his ideas, though, as we have seen earlier, most people in the field credit Krugman with pioneering the vaccine research and inspiring the commercial researchers who developed the first licensed hepatitis B vaccines.

Vaccine Design for Developing World Production

During the 1970s, while the pharmaceutical companies were busy on their hepatitis projects, Prince worked on his own version of the vaccine. His original motivation came directly out of his long-standing desire to prevent the disease. However, his research[3] and that of others soon made it clear that hepatitis was more severe and destructive in the

Third World than in the West. To fight hepatitis successfully, someone had to develop a technologically simple and cheap vaccine that could be directly transferred to the nations most severely affected. He knew that the drug companies working on the vaccine (e.g., Merck, Sharp & Dohme; Pasteur Vaccins) were using large and costly centrifuges, which made the process prohibitively expensive. The countries of Asia and Africa would not be able to afford such a costly technology.

Though Prince worked with both French and German pharmaceutical companies on his project, his goal was the transfer of the new technology from those firms to Third World countries. Prince was committed to a basic egalitarianism that took for granted that Asians and Africans could and should acquire the skills necessary to produce the medical products they consumed. He was put off by the widespread belief, found even among scientists at the highest levels of international health organizations, that quality vaccines could never be produced outside of America and Western Europe. He felt that such attitudes were little more than a continuation of the colonial mentality: a new variation of the "white man's burden," superficially cloaked under claims of practicality and scientific objectivity.

Prince's desire to develop his own vaccine became urgent when the Merck hepatitis B vaccine was licensed in the early 1980s at a cost of more than $30 a dose (with three doses required). The price came as a shock to the entire public health community. Prince had known for some time that the price that Merck (and other manufacturers) would charge could not be cheap because of the elaborate technology they employed, but he never dreamt it would be so expensive. Clearly, the Merck price meant that the vaccine would never be used in the countries where the disease caused the most devastation. Prince felt it would be "a rich man's vaccine and a poor man's disease." Prince was incensed that the price was inflated far above what even an expensive technology demanded.[4]

Inevitably, Prince's innate skepticism about the willingness or ability of most profit-oriented companies to meet basic human needs was strongly reinforced by the Merck pricing policy. What he had been trying to do up to then was simply create a cheap and uncomplicated technology that would enable the manufacturer to produce an affordable vaccine. After Merck priced its vaccine, Prince realized that in addition to controlling the cost of production, he had to be concerned with restraining the drug companies from seeking excessive profits. He wanted a "poor man's vaccine" that would not be limited to the upper and middle classes of the Third World. In addition, Prince wanted the transfer of vaccine technology to help build the industrial infrastructures of developing countries. He rejected the idea that such goals were outside the purview of scientists and better left to politicians and social planners.

The vaccine that he created met his goals. The production process of his plasma-derived vaccine was far simpler and cheaper than that of the vaccines others were developing. Even better, it used a flash heat purification method, which markedly increased the immunizing potency of the vaccine, as opposed to the chemical purification processes used elsewhere, which weakened the vaccine. Small doses of the vaccine produced by Prince's procedure were as effective as the much larger doses required with other vaccines. His vaccine required a substantially smaller amount of the most expensive ingredient, the blood of chronic carriers. For example, 10,000 to 20,000 doses of vaccine could be produced from one liter of highly infected plasma, whereas the Dutch Red Cross vaccine (a relatively inexpensive alternative) could produce only a tiny fraction of this number of doses from the same amount of blood.[5]

Henry Wilde, M.D., an outside observer who visited most of the chief vaccine manufacturers in the mid-1980s, assessed the hepatitis B vaccine situation as follows:

It appears that plasma-derived hepatitis vaccine has been developed by [a number of companies in the world]. . . . Their product is high technology and super-safety oriented without regard to cost-effectiveness or applicability to the developing world. They only realized later that the real need for hepatitis vaccine is in the poor countries of Asia and Africa. . . . Drug companies with new products are also not known for their altruism and have a track record of "charging what the traffic will bear" until competition enters the marketplace. . . . The only present plasma-derived process that was developed with the developing countries in mind appears to be the one of Dr. A[lfred] Prince.[6]

An Asian Commercial Partner and Production Technology Transfer

With the successful laboratory development of the vaccine, Prince needed a commercial partner to produce it on a massive scale. Both his German and French backers had pulled out for one reason or another. At that point, the early 1980s, a major opportunity presented itself in the person of Shin Seung-il, Ph.D., one of the new breed of academic scientists who became private entrepreneurs.

Shin was a professor of genetics at Albert Einstein Medical Center in New York City. He was a Korean-American with strong cultural and affectional ties to his original homeland. He and a group of other expatriate academicians had formed the Korean Bio-Science Club of New York as an informal discussion group in the early 1980s. In 1982 they unofficially created a non-profit group called Eugene Tech International (Eugene Tech), designed to provide scientific assistance to the government and academic institutions of Korea. This group wanted to share the expertise they had acquired in the United States to aid the technological advancement of their native land. At this point there appeared to be no conflict between their idealism and their desire to participate in the worldwide movement of academics into venture capitalism. Shin, representing this six-man group, negotiated with Samsung, the giant Korean conglomerate, to form a new group in the New York area that would provide laboratory training for visiting Korean scientists and do technology assessment for Samsung.[7] The problem for Shin was finding the best initial project with which to start the collaboration.

Since Eugene Tech had been founded largely as an expression of idealism—to aid the people of Korea in the modernizing process—it was not surprising that Shin was attracted to the problem of hepatitis. In Korea hepatitis B was a severe endemic problem. The country had a high percentage of chronic carriers, and hepatitis B–associated liver cancer was one of the most common cancers among Korean men.[8] The Merck vaccine was far too expensive to be used widely in Korea. Shin knew that the Korean government was engaged in a large-scale public health campaign to alert the population about the dangers of hepatitis, so what was clearly needed was an affordable Korean vaccine. A vaccine project would simultaneously be both good business and a socially progressive project. In addition, the humanitarian aspects of the venture would assist Samsung in building its corporate image. Eugene Tech proceeded to identify these factors to Samsung officials and specifically recommended the hepatitis project to the leadership of Cheil Sugar Company, a Samsung subsidiary that wished to expand into the biotechnology field. Cheil then set up a research and development laboratory in Korea to develop both biotechnology and pharmaceuticals.

A friend of Shin knew Prince and his work in developing a hepatitis B vaccine. At a meeting with Prince in the early 1980s, Shin proposed that the NYBC, Eugene Tech, and Cheil Sugar jointly develop the vaccine on an industrial production scale. They all agreed that they wanted a crash program that would get the vaccine out onto the market in record time.

The Korean Vaccine: Opportunities and Risks

For Prince, the agreement with the Koreans opened up the possibility of achieving all his major goals. He would be demonstrating the feasibility of transferring hepatitis B vaccine technology to a developing country, and his process would allow the vaccine to be sold for as little as $1 a dose, rather than the $30 or $40 that Merck was charging.

However, while the Cheil Sugar venture offered great possibilities, Prince realized that he would have to prod and push any private company to get a public-oriented result. Otherwise, "bottom-line" thinking would overwhelm the humanitarian aspects of the project.

Though the Cheil vaccine was Prince's "baby," he found that he could not afford the luxury of being an indulgent father. On many occasions Prince let the Korean pharmaceutical concern know that "I feel that I must share with you my serious concern with the progress of the HBV [hepatitis B virus] vaccine project."[9] He was anxious that the vaccine meet the recommendations and guidelines regarding purity and number of inactivation steps of the World Health Organization (WHO).[10] He protested that "there seems to me to be an excessive concentration on achieving licensing in the relatively limited Korean market, and a consequent weakening of our chances for acceptance on a worldwide basis,"[11] where the vaccine was so desperately needed.

For Prince, his vaccine would be significant only if it were available to the developing world, not just Korea. He felt he had to intervene when narrow business considerations threatened the usefulness of the whole project. For example, he wrote Shin that "I now understand that the basis for Cheil's reluctance to expand the vaccine effort is the assumption that the market for a plasma derived vaccine can last only for another two years or so,"[12] and thus was considered not worth too much investment. Such a narrow attitude threatened the viability of the venture. Prince believed that the new high-technology recombinant DNA vaccines, which Cheil feared would soon be on the market, would sell for more than plasma vaccines for at least a decade. The Cheil vaccine could be sold for as little as $1 or $1.50 a dose.[13] Indeed, given its high potency,[14] when manufactured in large quantities it might sell for as even low as $0.50 a dose. Such prices were mandatory if mass immunization projects were to be possible in the developing world. Recombinant DNA vaccines would be too expensive.[15]

Continuing Price and Technical Problems with the Koreans

To make the commercial vaccine the best it could be, Prince in 1985 helped put together a prestigious Clinical Trials Advisory Committee comprised of himself, Dr. R. Palmer Beasley (whose prospective study in Taiwan convinced the scientific community that hepatitis B was intimately linked to the development of primary liver cancer), and Dr. Cladd Stevens of the NYBC. He also involved scientists of world renown, such as Dr. James Maynard of the Centers for Disease Control (CDC), Dr. Xu Xi-Yi of Shanghai, China, and Dr. E. A. Ayoola of Nigeria to make sure the vaccine was up to world standards. (Later, most of these people would become members of the International Task Force).

When Prince realized that even outside experts did not guarantee a high quality of vaccine, he protested to Shin that

I am concerned that there is presently no continued effort in research and development to further improve the present Cheil vaccine. Certainly some work must be underway at Cheil, however, to the best of my knowledge this is not led by scientists experienced in this field.[16]

Prince had to deal not only with this problem but also with a more pervasive one emanating from the national culture in which Cheil was embedded. Korea did not have a strong clinical trial tradition; instead, it functioned the way German science had in the 1920s: "Herr Doktor Professor" said it was good or bad. Conducting a trial would be an insult to the established authority. Both Cheil and its chief competitor, the Korean Green Cross Corporation (KGCC), suffered from this problem.[17] In fact, KGCC had conducted even weaker trials than the researchers at Cheil, who had had the aid of Prince, Maynard, and Stevens. Whereas this shortcoming did not mean that the vaccine was ineffective, the trial data on dosage and other variables were not well enough supported as far as Prince was concerned, and he had to keep pressing them on this issue.

When Cheil decided to market the vaccine in Korea at prices ranging between $5 and $8 a dose, Prince felt the cost was simply out of line with both the needs of the developing world and the potential of the manufacturing process he had pioneered. Privately, and in association with others, he tried to persuade Cheil to lower the price. In October 1984 Cheil hosted a meeting in Seoul, South Korea, on immunization and the developing world. It was one of the first meetings concerned with the problem of getting hepatitis B vaccine to the Third World. Both Prince and Maynard pressured the company to agree to sell the vaccine to the public sector for $1 a dose. Cheil could make its profit by simultaneously selling to the private sector at whatever the market would bear. Prince and Maynard (and later the Task Force) continued to pressure Cheil for two years.[18] Their constant demands provided legitimacy for Shin's own efforts to persuade his superiors that the price had to be lowered. (After the Task Force was formed, their arguments finally produced positive results.)

During the period the Task Force was in the process of formation (mid- to late 1986), Prince and Maynard protested to Shin that Cheil lacked both an aggressive policy toward marketing the vaccine and an overall strategy for making it available through affordable sales and technology transfer. They told Shin that they could be far more supportive of Cheil if it developed a clear policy to get the vaccine out to the rest of the world. They explicitly warned Shin that they would look elsewhere for a manufacturer to support if the company did not change its ways.[19] For Prince, the goal was always to fight the hepatitis B pandemic successfully. The Cheil vaccine was only an instrument to that end; if it did not do the job, it was expendable.

The proof of where Prince's priorities lay was revealed after he (and by implication the Task Force that he then headed) was attacked by Western pharmaceutical companies for being too closely identified with Cheil. Since his goal was not personal financial gain, he promptly renounced all of his royalty rights as the vaccine's developer. As we will see later, the intense level of conflict and hostility that characterizes the often "brutal"[20] politics of international health is such that this action did not deter critics from continuing to impugn his motives and objectivity. Prince's opponents continued to wage a war of rumor and innuendo against him and the group that he led.

By the time the International Task Force on Hepatitis B Immunization was formed, Prince had been working on an inexpensive and effective vaccine for more than ten years. He had expended his efforts on effectively combating the disease both in the laboratory and in the outside world. He had developed a vaccine that was cheap and uncomplicated enough to make the mass immunization of children in the Third World a real possibility. If hepatitis B could be avoided and the carrier stage eliminated, not only would one of the world's most widespread viral diseases be eradicated, but the epidemic of liver cancer in developing countries would cease as well. Such a result would constitute the most important victory ever achieved in the war against cancer.

In addition to developing an affordable vaccine and finding a manufacturer for it, Prince had forged informal links with key scientists from around the world (James Maynard, R. Palmer Beasley, Xu Xi-Yi, and E. A. Ayoola) who shared his goals and would later help to make the Task Force an effective agent for lobbying the world health community. The development of Prince's "Third World vaccine" was initially the indispensable element necessary for the creation of the International Task Force on Hepatitis B Immunization.

James Maynard

James Maynard, M.D., Ph.D., was the head of the Hepatitis Branch of the CDC in Atlanta, Georgia. In that capacity, during much of the 1970s and into the early 1980s, he probably was the most important public health official in the world dealing with hepatitis problems. The CDC, along with WHO, was the focal point for those concerned with matters of international health. Since people from around the world looked to Atlanta as well as Geneva for aid in dealing with their problems, both served a multinational constituency. However, in dealing with hepatitis B, the CDC's human and financial resources were far greater than those of WHO.

Maynard was especially drawn to international health issues. He was of Canadian parentage and originally thought of seeking his future in Canada, but he was advised that he would not find enough opportunity there. If he was interested in the world arena he would have to work in the United States, and in America the biggest stage was provided by the CDC.[21]

Maynard's vision of himself as a public servant was the antithesis of that normally associated with government employees. He did not waste his or his subordinates' time on wasteful bureaucratic paperwork. His goal was to understand the hepatitises (A, B, C, D, and E) scientifically and do whatever was necessary to control their spread. He and his people were dedicated to conducting the best laboratory work, undertaking the most useful epidemiological research, and helping devise the most effective disease control programs that could be implemented.[22] He was determined not to allow red tape to interfere with achieving those goals. In pursuit of his objectives he helped get his subgroup at CDC recognized as a WHO Collaborating Centre for Hepatitis. He brought together a top-quality staff with assistants who were good enough to free him from the burden of daily oversight, enabling him to devote more of his time to working in the international arena. He became one of the key experts on whom WHO came to rely in dealing with hepatitis problems anywhere in the world. He also served as one of WHO's chief advisers in setting WHO's biological standards for hepatitis B vaccines after those vaccines became available.

Maynard's Guiding Philosophy

Like Prince, Maynard has had a philosophical commitment to working for the public good, independent of private marketplace considerations. Perhaps because of his roots in Canada, where democratic socialism has not been a dirty word or an oxymoron, he has believed that government can and must meet the needs of its people in a way that capitalistic enterprises cannot. Even today, despite his pleasure at the collapse of pseudo-socialism in the Soviet bloc, he has not been happy with the chest-thumping of those conservative Americans who claim that laissez-faire capitalism has been proven the best and only viable way to run human societies. He sees such self-congratulation as just a passing conceit, a result of the pendulum "over-swinging" once again in the perennial competition between the public and private sectors. He believes such self-satisfaction will end when capitalism once again demonstrates that on its own it cannot adequately meet basic human needs. Certainly, says Maynard, the drug companies, designed as they are for maximum profits rather than for finding cures for people, will not work for the public good in the absence of external pressure. He sees government as an indispensable participant because of its ability to produce and distribute biologics that people need but which the private sector ignores.[23]

One of the key advantages of his position at the CDC was the large degree of autonomy the organization allowed him as a member of its senior staff. Maynard had almost total discretion in the allocation of the official budget of the Hepatitis Branch. He did not have to go "up-stairs" to have key activities approved. As Maynard put it, once the CDC leadership had confidence in a person, they allowed him or her a great deal of freedom. Individuals who made mistakes could lose their autonomy, but the leadership corrected them only after the fact. There were political pressures in controversial areas like AIDS research and family planning that limited independent action; the more the contro-versy, the more oversight from higher levels. Fortunately, according to Maynard, hepatitis B was not in the public spotlight, and those re-straints did not apply to him.

Because of his relative freedom over the Hepatitis Branch, not only was Maynard able to devote much of his own time to working in the international arena, but he could call on the assistance of key members of his staff to investigate problems, do research, and write proposals for developing countries. In matters relating to hepatitis B on the interna-tional level, Maynard was the CDC personified. He brought with him an aura of great power and influence.

Focus on Affordable Mass Immunization Programs in the Developing World

One of the places Maynard wished to have an effect was in Thailand. The Thais, along with most Southeast Asians, had a major hepatitis B problem. Wearing both the hat of Chief of the CDC's Hepatitis Branch and that of WHO Expert Consultant, Maynard advocated a Thai National Hepatitis B Immunization Program in the early 1980s. He wanted to get the U.S. Agency for International Development (USAID) to fund part of the immunization work through a bilateral agreement with the Thais.[24] He hoped that the Thais could begin with a model program in a selected part of the country. Such a project would demonstrate the feasibility of a nationwide campaign and help prove that hepatitis could be successfully integrated into the Thai Expanded Programme for Immunization (EPI).[25] Maynard felt that he could work to bring together the various Thai organizations and individuals needed to create a demonstration project. He believed that the American CDC could successfully act as a catalyst for the creation of such models. Once created, the models would inspire not only the host country (Thailand) but other developing countries as well.[26] In fact, it could help persuade the head of WHO's EPI that hepatitis B should be adopted as the seventh universal vaccine, and thus be made available to all the world's poor children.

In his attempts to create a model project in Thailand, Maynard became familiar with the health politics of that nation. One of his first goals was to get the Ministry of Public Health to assist in raising the priority given hepatitis B in relation to other diseases. He found himself frustrated by the large size of the Ministry's Hepatitis Committee (approximately twenty members), each member of which represented a different vested interest. Even when the committee could manage to meet, they rarely agreed upon even the simplest issues.[27] (The Task Force later adopted Maynard's "model project" concept and carried it out much more effectively than Maynard had been able to do acting on his own.)

Maynard, like Prince, was committed to the idea of a cheap vaccine, the technology of which could be transferred to developing countries. He started from premises very similar to those of Prince. Maynard knew the problem of getting an affordable vaccine was especially acute in the developing world. The only way to get reasonably priced hepatitis B vaccines was to encourage competition, whether the companies wanted it or not—a motivating role he felt the CDC could and should play. Maynard believed that the more producers involved, the greater the competition would be.[28] He looked favorably upon developing countries producing their own health products, both as a matter of national pride and as a way of building their economic infrastructures. Like Prince, he disagreed with those who saw quality vaccine production as a natural and inevitable monopoly of the West and Japan. Maynard was vehemently opposed to the rigidity of WHO's Biological Standard for Hepatitis B Vaccines, which he felt was unnecessarily restrictive, harmful to vaccine potency, and almost impossible for Third World producers to meet.[29]

The Prince Vaccine and Hepatitis B in the Third World

After the Prince vaccine became commercially available in 1982, Maynard quickly became convinced that universal childhood vaccination rather than selective high-risk immunization was the only way to combat and ultimately to eradicate the scourge of hepatitis B. It was clear to him that even in low endemicity countries such as the United States, only universal vaccination would have any significant effect. The need for universal vaccination was even greater in high endemicity countries in the developing world.[30]

Maynard could champion the idea of universal vaccination programs in the developing world[31] not only because he believed that any other, more limited program would fail, but also because he believed that the price of the vaccine could be brought down enough for mass immunization. It was his belief, as it was Prince's, that the price of the vaccine had little relationship to its cost of manufacture. Despite claims by Merck and others that the vaccine was very expensive to produce, Maynard knew that the French producer, Pasteur Vaccins, was shipping bulk vaccine to Taiwan for as low as $4 per shot.[32]

Maynard was so upset by the price that Merck was charging that he coined the term "boutique vaccine" to characterize the absurdity of the situation. He and one of his key staff members, Mark Kane, M.D., completed a study in 1983 which showed that the vaccine would have to sell for $1 a dose or less to be usable in the EPI[33] and in mass immunization campaigns. He believed that this low price was realistic, and he became a vocal proponent of the $1-a-dose concept at WHO hepatitis B international meetings. In that capacity he came up against the hostility of such powerful men as Frank Perkins, M.D., head of Biologics at WHO, who promoted the view that quality vaccines could only be produced in the United States and Western Europe.[34]

Maynard heard from many vaccine researchers that new, cheap vaccines were on the verge of being produced (one researcher at Connaught in Canada told him that a mammalian cell–derived recombinant DNA vaccine would cost $1 a dose,[35] and Dr. Kenneth Macintosh at the Federal Drug Administration said the FDA was talking of producing a $1-a-dose vaccine itself).[36] However, Prince's plasma-derived vaccine was the only one actually out on the market. Maynard was deeply impressed with the vaccine's potential and was willing to aid Prince in making sure that it was good enough and cheap enough to make the goal of mass immunization a reality; he helped design trials to test and perfect the Cheil vaccine.

As Chief of the CDC's Hepatitis Branch, Maynard was in an excellent position to provide legitimacy for the fledgling Cheil vaccine. For example, in 1985, at a time when Cheil was struggling to overcome unexpected obstacles to obtaining licensure in Korea, Maynard visited Seoul and made a strong appeal on behalf of Cheil's innovative heat-inactivation technique. He praised its economy, efficiency, and safety.[37]

Speaking as a ranking CDC official, he had a powerful effect in Korean scientific and governmental circles. On another occasion in the mid-1980s, when the leadership of the Oswaldo Cruz Institute in Brazil wrote the CDC to ask for guidance in gaining access to the Prince/NYBC technology, Maynard enthusiastically worked to transfer the technology to Brazil.

In 1985, when an American non-profit organization (Program for Appropriate Technology in Health) asked his advice on choosing the best vaccine to transfer to the developing world, he responded that both the Merck and Prince vaccines were workable, but the NYBC and Korean producers supplying the latter vaccine would be more flexible and respond more rapidly to demands. Their process was specifically designed for developing countries. He placed great emphasis on the speed (nine months) with which the Korean factory had been set up[38] and contrasted it favorably to what he called Merck's "fiasco" in transferring hepatitis B technology to Singapore.[39]

Maynard's commitment to mass immunization against hepatitis B, his favorable view of the Prince vaccine, and his pivotal position at the CDC made it possible for him to aid significantly the movement toward an affordable vaccine. The personal and professional links he had formed with Prince would provide a firm foundation for their later collaboration on the Task Force. However, his championing of the Prince/Cheil product would open him up to personal attacks on his objectivity. Those attacks would plague Maynard, Prince, and ultimately the organization they would help create.

Ian Gust

In the years before the formation of the International Task Force on Hepatitis B Immunization, one of Maynard's most important activities outside the United States was his work in the creation of the WHO's Western Pacific Regional Office (WPRO) Task Force on Hepatitis B. In many ways the WPRO group served as the model for the later Task Force.

The inspiration for the WPRO Task Force came from Ian Gust, M.D., an Australian virologist.[40] Gust, like Prince and Maynard, was a man dedicated to the ideal of an active public sector that addressed human needs. He traced his personal commitment to the well-being of the common man back to the socialism of his working-class Polish-Jewish father.

Gust and Maynard decided in the late 1970s that they should work on the hepatitis B problem in Asia, using the resources available through WPRO. More than 150 million chronic carriers of the virus lived in the countries served by WPRO.[41] Of these people, fully 40 percent of the male carriers and 20 percent of the female carriers would ultimately die from the consequences of chronic hepatitis B virus infection. Gust graphically presented the human meaning behind these statistics at an early hepatitis B conference:

On the basis of [persuasive] . . . data, we can calculate that every minute, a child is born who will die of the long-term sequelae of hepatitis B. To put this into perspective, in the time between my leaving Melbourne on Friday and arriving home on Tuesday morning, 5,400 children will have been born who are condemned to die from one of the sequelae of chronic hepatitis B infection (cirrhosis, chronic active hepatitis, primary hepatocellular carcinoma).[42]

Gust and Maynard obtained the cooperation of Umenai Takusai, M.D.,[43] Regional Advisor for Communicable Diseases for WPRO. He in turn was influential with his compatriot, Nakajima Hiroshi, M.D., Ph.D., who headed the office. With their cooperation WPRO "organized a series of meetings and seminars to educate scientists, and health officials, . . . train laboratory workers and . . . support . . . collaborative studies . . . aimed at defining the prevalence and the incidence of serious sequelae."[44] In 1981 the WHO Western Pacific Advisory Committee on Medical Research received a report on hepatitis B and convened an experts' meeting. The experts recommended that WHO develop programs for control of hepatitis B, and suggested that the Regional Director should support efforts to stimulate production and distribution of high-quality diagnostic reagents and should encourage studies aimed at prevention of the carrier state. Their report urged him to take advantage of WHO Collaborating Centres in the region to train scientists to provide expert advice and organize research projects and identified three laboratories in the region (Tokyo Metropolitan Institute of Medical Science, Nagaski Chuo Hospital, and Fairfield Hospital in Melbourne) to assist in the process. The experts also encouraged member countries to assign national hepatitis laboratories to collect and transmit epidemiologic data, as well as to produce working reagents and develop local training programs.[45]

To emphasize its commitment and provide a focal point for activities, WPRO set up a Task Force on Hepatitis B in 1983. It was the first WHO regional task force anywhere in the world. The major thrust of the WPRO program was to encourage self-sufficiency in reagent and vaccine production among all its member nations. One of the most important results of WPRO activity was the education of regional leaders as to the importance of the hepatitis B pandemic:

From the Regional Director down, staff of the Regional Office and members of the Task Force have taken a high profile. By arranging meetings, workshops, publications and most importantly discussions with policy-makers, we have tried to convince politicians that HB [hepatitis B] is a problem worth controlling and that the tools to achieve it are now available.[46]

WPRO collected information on the degree of the hepatitis B problem in different countries and on its various modes of transmission. The Task Force then helped governments decide on the different types of vaccine they needed. It suggested ways to meet local needs, for example, by buying vaccine, making it, or collecting infected plasma locally and shipping it to collection centers abroad, where it could be processed into vaccine and sent back. It also helped local authorities decide if high-risk or universal immunization was the best strategy for them.

In an attempt to maximize its effectiveness, the WPRO Task Force went directly to the Ministries of Health in the various countries. The Task Force felt that the top leaders had to be approached first, and it was able to visit the Ministers of Health under WHO auspices. These activities required a significant amount of lobbying, which proved to be very successful. The high point of the WPRO Task Force was the groundbreaking transfer of hepatitis B vaccine technology from the developed world to the People's Republic of China.

WPRO and the Opening of China

Gust and Maynard found a rare "window of opportunity"[47] for their pioneering work against hepatitis B. That opportunity developed due to the personality of the WPRO Regional Director, Nakajima, and as a result of the national politics within WHO.

Nakajima was an ambitious man determined to make his mark on the world, and the leadership of WPRO was a good place to begin. His goal was to create a reputation for himself that would ultimately lead to the WHO Director-Generalship in Geneva. He was primed to prove himself with an innovative and spectacular problem-solving project.

Nakajima was also a Japanese national. WHO allocates staff positions based upon the contribution each nation makes toward its budget. Japan, given its financial contribution, was significantly under-represented, making Nakajima, as a high-ranking Japanese WHO official, especially prominent and important. Representatives of different countries often given special attention to the interests of their respective homelands.[48] Ideally the interests of the individual's nation of origin and the goals of WHO will coincide, though this is not always the case. Japan's overseas assistance programs have emphasized health and agriculture. At the same time, Japan's industrial products have been of superior quality. Thus, the interests of WHO in meeting health needs and the interests of the Japanese in providing assistance (and creating future markets) have complemented each other.[49]

One of the major goals of both WHO and Japan was to "open" China to the outside world: The Japanese wanted to enhance the rapprochement between the two countries; WHO wanted to generate significant interaction between China and WHO. A WPRO project that could simultaneously serve the interests of WHO, Japan, and China would be a major personal triumph for Nakajima. It did not have to be hepatitis B—some other project would have done the job just as well—but the opportunity was there, and Gust's and Maynard's initiative fit the needs of all the concerned parties.[50] As Maynard said, it was vital "to be sensitive to the political currents that allow . . . us to act for health,"[51] and he and Gust were masters of such diplomacy:

> China was seen as the key; the Japanese were very interested in wooing the Chinese. Mass immunization was a good way to do that. So we [on the WPRO Task Force] made China our key [too]. We created interest and expectations in [the area of] immunization. . . . Now we needed to get vaccine in large quantities at a good price. Without alternative supplies it was not possible. We felt encouraging local production was the key. We did not know how—we did not care if it was a big guy with a local subsidiary, or a local guy or [just] plasma from a country sent out [and returned from a processing laboratory in another country]. . . . China wanted a transfer of technology [and it had] . . . strong support from Nakajima and the Japanese government. We helped the Chinese to produce their own vaccine.[52]

To transfer the technology to China, Maynard, Gust, Umenai, Nakajima, and two Japanese scientists engaged in "Kissinger-style" shuttling to and from China.[53] All told, the transfer entailed 50 to 100 visits by consultants over a five-year period.[54] Nakajima arranged for Japan's Kitasato Institute to give the technology to China essentially cost-free, and he raised the money for this venture from Agfund (Arab Gulf Fund, a WHO donor).[55] For the Japanese the transfer was a form of foreign assistance which helped establish a good reputation for Japanese products and technology in China.[56] China set up five different vaccine-producing centers and by 1991 had produced twenty-two million doses of vaccine.

The Real but Limited Success of the WPRO Task Force

For Gust and Maynard, the WPRO Task Force was in many ways a gratifying success. It was the boldest attack on hepatitis B anywhere in the world. All of its accomplishments had been achieved at little or no cost. No new buildings or organizations had been created, and WHO had kept its monetary contribution to a symbolic level. Nevertheless, WHO's official support had helped scientists obtain money from their own governments. In addition, WHO's influence was important in altering national priorities and favorably influencing the allocation of the funds of international agencies to the hepatitis B problem. Especially important was the approach: "The key to the success of the Task Force [was] . . . working with and through the agency of local organizations, a process which t[ook] time and patience,"[57] but which paid off handsomely. As Gust put it:

International agencies such as WHO are sometimes criticized for their inability to translate good intentions into practical achievements. [The WPRO Task Force was an excellent example of] how WHO can act as a catalyst to bring scientists and public health authorities together.[58]

However, despite the many successes of the WPRO effort, there were significant problems. Most important, the China hepatitis B vaccine technology transfer, the jewel in the crown of the Task Force's work, was seriously flawed.

The Chinese established five different centers for vaccine production, but the mechanisms they used to set them up and to distribute their product were all faulty. Universal childhood vaccination, the goal of the transfer, was not achieved because not enough of the vaccine could be produced. What they did produce they did not effectively distribute.

In part, hepatitis B vaccine manufacturing became a victim of China's movement to privatize pharmaceutical and health care services. It was the first "baby vaccine" that was not provided free of charge to all Chinese children. The production centers needed more money from the government to increase their efficiency and quality. Instead, the money came in the form of a loan from the Bank of China. Costs had to be met by charging a higher price than most rural Chinese could afford. In addition, with the privatization of health delivery, the "barefoot" doctor was abolished and became the village doctor. Instead of getting a monthly salary, he or she became an entrepreneur who had to be paid for giving any new vaccine. Thus the vaccine sat on the shelf for lack of an effective market. In addition to these unfortunate changes, the vaccine manufacturing centers experienced major problems in production which reduced the efficacy and consistency of the vaccine, significantly impeding the fight against the epidemic.[59]

Even the successes were not good enough as far as Gust was concerned. By 1986 it became clear to him that "despite the lead being taken in the Western Pacific, little was being done to address hepatitis B immunization in other developing areas of the world."[60] There were many reasons for this unacceptable situation: differences in strength among WHO regional offices, the lack of local expertise, different health care systems, political instability, lack of interest by local authorities, and the high cost of the vaccine.[61] Because of these feelings, both Gust and Maynard were ready for some larger venture.

Maynard, along with R. Palmer Beasley, the scientist whose work established the link between hepatitis B and liver cancer, tried to get WHO in Geneva to set up a general task force to focus on hepatitis B. At one of the 1985 Global Advisory Group meetings, they made a formal recommendation that WHO designate a full-time employee to be responsible for tracking hepatitis B immunization programs around the world. Dr. Fakhry Assaad, WHO's Director of the Division of Communicable Diseases, refused to implement the recommendation.[62]

Richard Mahoney

At that point a deus ex machina entered the hepatitis picture: the deus went by the name of Richard Mahoney, Ph.D., and his machina was a nonprofit organization called Program for Appropriate Technology in Health (PATH), headquartered in Seattle, Washington.

Mahoney was a very different kind of person from Prince, Maynard, or Gust. The latter three were dedicated public servants, long concerned with the scientific and social problems surrounding the hepatitis B pandemic. They had strong moral and ideological commitments to addressing human needs and deep suspicions that private enterprise was inherently incapable of achieving that goal. They were, however, unfamiliar with the actual workings of the private sector.

While Mahoney's career was situated in philanthropic and nonprofit organizations, these institutions were usually supported directly or indirectly by the fruits of corporate profits, so he gained in-depth knowledge and broad respect for the ability of private enterprise to generate innovative, quality goods and services. He was suspicious of bureaucratic inefficiency and ineptitude and was skeptical of government's ability to produce or distribute products of high quality. Compared with the jaundiced eye that Prince, Maynard, and Gust cast toward business, Mahoney's attitude was friendly and collaborative.

Nevertheless, his pro-business attitude was tempered by his keen awareness of the private sector's commitment to the bottom line and of the propensity for profit-hunger to take precedence over the common good. He was no Pollyanna about the relationship between business and the public interest. He strongly believed that people, the poor as well as the rich, inherently deserved to have their needs adequately served, but he concluded that the best way to do that was to harness and then channel business energies in ways that modified the profit motive rather than dispensed with it.

Mahoney combined an entrepreneurial spirit with an idealistic goal. He was always searching for new worlds to conquer, new problems to solve, and new fields in which to make his mark. Where private entrepreneurs sought profits and power, Mahoney pursued philanthropic accomplishments, prestige, and reputation with the same hunger. He harnessed his own ambitions so that they worked for the common good, and he sought to yoke private enterprise for the same goal. He created in himself a model for the possibility and necessity of socializing and humanizing entrepreneurial ambition.

Mahoney and PATH Form a Powerful Team

PATH, the organization that Mahoney represented, was likewise a dynamo of enterprise. The same world-conquering ambition that motivated Mahoney strongly motivated PATH. This organization also harnessed and channeled its basically aggressive entrepreneurial spirit into more socially responsible forms. For example, to guarantee that PATH did not drift far from its goal of meeting the needs of the developing world, its board of directors was composed exclusively of individuals from Third World countries.[63]

The coming together of men like Prince, Maynard, and Gust with Mahoney and PATH, if not quite a marriage of opposites, was nevertheless in spirit, outlook, and temperament an unusual union. It was also a historic occasion. While the three scientists were major figures in the infectious disease community, at this juncture Mahoney was the "indispensable man." It was Mahoney who transformed the forces fighting the hepatitis B pandemic from a collection of able guerrilla leaders into an effective, organized army.

Mahoney and PATH were latecomers to the war against hepatitis B. PATH's official mission was to help developing nations gain access to the best and cheapest technology available to meet their health needs. This did not mean "bamboo technology [or] how to make stoves out of old tin cans,"[64] but rather the identification and introduction of the most promising Western technology that would make a contribution to the quality of life. Sometimes the technology PATH chose was very sophisticated, sometimes very simple.[65]

Mahoney and PATH saw their role as a unique one because they were willing to serve as a bridge between the private and public sectors. If private companies were involved in health activities, PATH could work to insure that public sector needs were given adequate attention. On the other hand, if public organizations undertook a project, PATH could guarantee that the project would have access to the highest-quality methodology and management approaches—usually found only in the private sector.[66] PATH prided itself on being nonpolitical and nonideological; it was willing to lend assistance to public or private organizations and to cooperate with both capitalists and socialists. Most of the time PATH found that private sector companies could deliver quality products whereas state pharmaceutical factories could not. Accordingly, PATH usually recommended private companies, but it would work willingly with private or public groups and try to antici-pate and respond to any difficulties it found among both types of organizations.[67]

Since PATH's mandate was to find and help deliver appropriate technology in health, the organization was constantly looking for new challenges that would exercise and justify its talents as well as keep it funded. Before the hepatitis B project, its largest program was helping the Chinese government to upgrade and construct contraceptive pro-duction facilities. The lessons learned in China were transferable to other developing countries. Even more important, in an earlier Mexi-can project, PATH had pioneered and perfected skills that would prove invaluable in the Third World: the development of materials expressly for semiliterate and illiterate people; utilization of Focus Group Discussions in villages to discover what local people know about local problems; development of pictures rather than written texts to educate the public; and creation of "feedback" mechanisms that could help adjust the message when it did not work effectively.[68]

Awareness of the Hepatitis B Problem in Asia

The problem of hepatitis B was forced upon Mahoney's attention by two separate series of events during 1984. The first and most impor-tant influence came from Indonesia. During that year PATH received a large grant from USAID to work in establishing local production of health products. During a visit to the Minister of Health, Lyle Saun-ders, a PATH consultant, asked what activities PATH could undertake that would be most supportive of the objectives of the government. He was told that President Suharto had informed the Minister of Health that the President's friend and golf partner had died from liver cancer, and Suharto wanted something done about this all-too-common dis-ease. The Minister told Saunders he would be gratified if PATH could do something about hepatitis B, an agent closely associated with liver cancer. As Mahoney put it, when a Minister of Health specifically asks for help, PATH "jumps."[69] Since PATH's particular expertise was in the introduction and local manufacture of health products, the request was seen as compatible with its organizational mission.[70]

When the Indonesian request for aid was made, Mahoney did not even know the difference between hepatitis A and hepatitis B, but he quickly educated himself. In a meeting with the Minister of Health, Mahoney pointed out that there was a safe and effective vaccine for hepatitis B which would prevent liver cancer—frequently a long-term sequela of hepatitis virus infection. Mahoney also told him that local production of both the vaccine and hepatitis B diagnostics was possible. PATH had money to help set up local production when and if the government requested it. Since the Minister was enthusiastic about the idea of local vaccine production, PATH proceeded to do a feasibility study of the financial, technical, and management requirements for such a project.

PATH methodology in preparing a project has always begun with in-depth background research. This has included locating the best and most knowledgeable people on the subject and going to them no matter where they may be. PATH then intensively interviews each purported expert to elicit his or her view of the parameters of the problem and the various competing solutions. Afterward, each expert is used as a referral source for additional names of key people, products, or technology in the field. The opinions of each expert are then compared with those of individuals already interviewed until a clear picture of the various options is obtained. Once this is done, the best-quality and least expensive technology or product is located, and negotiations for obtaining or transferring its technology are undertaken. This process of mastering the field is time-consuming, intense, and expensive, but it has paid off for PATH.

While the main push toward involvement with hepatitis B came from Indonesia, a secondary influence came out of Thailand. Henry Wilde, M.D., a highly knowledgeable and perceptive American ex-foreign service officer in Thailand, was an advisor to PATH. According to Wilde, "Rich [Mahoney] had USAID technology transfer grants but did not know what to transfer. He had a list of possibilities. In Thailand pharmaceuticals were very efficient and cheap. They copied everything. I got on the vaccine track. . . . [M]y research interest was rabies."[71] And rabies seemed like a good issue for PATH. Thailand had a significant rabies problem, and the locally produced vaccine, derived from brain tissue, was of inferior quality and carried a high risk of death for users.[72] In researching the local scientific, governmental, and technical resources for upgrading the rabies vaccine production process, Mahoney and Wilde discovered that many academic and scientific individuals and groups wanted to deal with production of both rabies and hepatitis B vaccines. The two diseases were seen as important local problems that provided significant areas of opportunity for building a sophisticated Thai manufacturing infrastructure. The Thais saw hepatitis B vaccine production as naturally lending itself to a piggyback arrangement with any new rabies vaccine manufacturing facility.

Thus, hepatitis B was a pressing problem in both Indonesia and Thailand and provided a major opportunity for constructive intervention. Since PATH was "the new kid on the block" in these countries and wished to establish its credentials,[73] it needed something that was both new and exciting to get itself noticed. Hepatitis B vaccine development seemed to be the perfect proving ground. Even more important, the vaccine suggested to Mahoney a grand strategy and goal for his organization. He expressed his view in a letter to the President of PATH:

> It seemed to me there is the opportunity for PATH to become one of the central agencies in the new initiative to expand immunization programs in developing countries. Currently, WHO is undertaking research and supporting services; UNICEF is supporting service provision; USAID, The World Bank, and other donors are addressing themselves almost exclusively to public sector activities. No agency is addressing itself directly to stimulating and encouraging private sector involvement. . . . [T]his would seem a golden opportunity to match our capabilities and interest with what seems to be a major, unmet need in the efforts to expand immunization services to developing world people.[74]

No entrepreneurial empire builder could have been more ambitious. The beauty of focusing on hepatitis B was that Mahoney and PATH could serve the people of the Third World, fight a devastating disease, carry out PATH's idealistic organizational mission, be at the center of a pioneering health movement, make a big splash, and obtain funds, all at the same time. What better example of socially molded ambition could there be?

Mahoney Meets the Hepatitis Experts

As Mahoney and PATH searched for expert information on hepatitis B, he and other members of the staff met with Drs. Maurice Hilleman (the developer of the Merck vaccine), Robert Gerety of the FDA, Robert Purcell of the National Institutes of Health, James Maynard of the CDC, and representatives of such vaccine manufacturers as Pasteur Vaccins, Genentech, and the Dutch Red Cross.

At first Merck, the manufacturer of one of the two initially licensed plasma-derived hepatitis B vaccines and leader in the development of the second-generation recombinant DNA vaccines, looked like the most promising prospect. The government of Indonesia was interested in getting the newest and most sophisticated technology. Merck officials told Mahoney that the company did not see its new recombinant DNA vaccine as "adding to its bottom line but rather as a way to make public health contributions to the developing countries . . . [with] public relations benefits . . . outweigh[ing] any profits that might be made."[75] The lack of capital for technology transfer was also a major problem throughout the world. Merck's leadership saw PATH's USAID-funded project (called Health Link) as a potential source of money for identifying capital resources and carrying out feasibility studies. Since Merck lacked the staffing necessary to permit the time investment for feasibility studies, PATH could fill that vital role. Merck went so far as to offer PATH the right to become its exclusive representative. A relationship with Merck was very attractive to Mahoney, at least initially.[76]

The possibility of working with Merck was considered viable for quite a while.[77] However, as more expert information came in, especially from interviews conducted by Wilde in Europe and America, Mahoney realized that recombinant DNA technology was too sophisticated and expensive to transfer to developing countries such as Thailand and Indonesia.

Conversations between a PATH representative and Maynard at the CDC supported a shift away from both Merck's recombinant DNA and its plasma-derived vaccine.[78] Maynard's extensive knowledge, well-argued positions, and high international reputation eventually made him a key PATH adviser on locating other potential vaccine sources. That Maynard was trying to organize a hepatitis B model project in Thailand and had close ties to key government officials there added to his attractiveness and persuasiveness. PATH and Maynard had many goals and interests in common, and PATH was enthusiastic about working with Maynard not only in Asia but also in Latin America.

PATH's interest in Maynard was increasingly matched by Maynard's interest in PATH. However, for Maynard to cooperate with PATH, it would have to defuse his initial suspicion of its involvement with the private sector. Once Maynard was convinced that PATH was primarily motivated by humanitarian concerns rather than private profit, he found collaboration an attractive possibility.[79]

Mahoney Learns of Prince's Vaccine

Early in his research activities Mahoney had heard of Alfred Prince and his Cheil vaccine. He elected to put off meeting with Prince, however, since he did not want to involve himself with someone associated with a commercial venture for fear Prince would be biased and unreliable.[80] Maynard, however, strongly testified to the integrity of both Prince and the NYBC and said that PATH could work with either Merck or NYBC, but that Merck would present more problems because the NYBC (with its Eugene Tech/Cheil Sugar vaccine) would be more flexible than the larger Merck.[81] In addition, NYBC was oriented more toward developing countries, whereas Merck had done poorly in its attempt to transfer hepatitis B vaccine technology to Singapore.[82] With Maynard's strong endorsement Mahoney met with Prince at the NYBC—where he also met with Shin Seung-il of Eugene Tech/Cheil Sugar.

The initial attraction of Prince and the NYBC for Mahoney was not their vaccine per se, but the fact that they knew about the production process. Maynard, for all his scientific expertise, did not have detailed information on the equipment, management, and machinery that were necessary to set up a plant:

> We did not want to go to private industry [for technical information]. If you go to them then you must tell them it is only academic or you . . . [are willing to have them] be the supplier. We did not want either one. . . . Prince allowed us to get around this. He hadn't set up a factory himself, but he worked on setting up the Korean factory. . . . Prince's cheap vaccine was [initially an] added feature. But the key was he knew what machinery you need, what manpower, etc.— though he did not know all [the] things [we needed to know].[83]

Mahoney found both Prince and Shin of Eugene Tech/Cheil Sugar to be very sympathetic to PATH's ideas, especially its concern for aid to developing countries. Mahoney spent a lot of time with Shin and found him surprisingly cooperative, willing to share far more technical information about establishing a vaccine factory than were scientists affiliated with other private companies. Mahoney also discovered that Prince had successfully convinced the Cheil leadership of the fundamental importance of making the new vaccine affordable.[84] Mahoney was increasingly convinced that the Prince/Cheil vaccine was the best vaccine for PATH to transfer to Asia: it was a relatively simple and inexpensive production process, and the vaccine was cheap, safe, and potent. Cheil looked promising not only for Indonesia but also (at some future time) for Thailand.

The NYBC was also attractive to PATH. NYBC conducted original research and brought products to the prototypic stage of development, but it did not have the marketing and licensing capacity to commercialize its innovations. It was in some ways an internationally oriented organization, but it was primarily focused on the local New York City community. NYBC's lack of entrepreneurial skills raised the possibility of fruitful collaboration between PATH and NYBC. Such cooperation would aid the mission of both institutions.[85] Prince expressed the hope that at some point the NYBC itself would manufacture his vaccine for export to the Latin American and African markets (areas not included in the Cheil license). Mahoney envisioned the possibility of providing a loan to the NYBC, not so much to finance such a venture but rather to establish a formal relationship between PATH and the NYBC that could lead to further activities in the future.[86]

At this point (1985) PATH prepared a report for the Indonesian Minister of Health.[87] The study informed him that local vaccine production was feasible but that the recombinant DNA vaccine was not a viable choice.[88] Instead, a plasma-derived vaccine offered the best possibilities for Indonesia. The report also recommended to the Minister the usefulness of the NYBC/Cheil vaccine. In fact, it suggested that he visit Korea and meet personally with the Cheil personnel. The Minister responded favorably to the suggestion about the NYBC, but he expressed his desire to avoid working directly with the Koreans. In the Minister's estimation, the NYBC carried considerable prestige, while Korean companies lacked a favorable reputation. The Minister believed that the Koreans, as good businessmen, would understand that they needed to be "invisible" in any arrangement that was reached.[89] The Minister told PATH that he wanted to visit the NYBC after he attended an international meeting in Geneva. Mahoney suggested that while he was in the New York area he also visit Merck and, later, PATH headquarters in Seattle and Cheil Sugar in Korea.[90]

While PATH was dealing with the Minister of Health, it was also in contact with leading Indonesian businessmen who imported or produced vaccines. Cheil Sugar wanted to quickly establish a distribution arrangement with one of these private entrepreneurs. However, the Indonesian businessmen, like the Minister of Health, wanted the Korean connection hidden.[91]

During the last months of 1985 PATH was deeply involved in attempting to introduce the Prince/Cheil vaccine into Indonesia—as the first step, it was hoped, in the transfer of technology for production of the hepatitis B vaccine. PATH persuaded Maynard to lend his prestige to help counteract the influence of Indonesian scientists and officials who insisted that only the most advanced vaccine technology (i.e., recombinant DNA techniques) and the biggest European/American manufacturers were good enough for Indonesia. For PATH it was absolutely vital that "Maynard . . . help blunt objections raised by [local people] . . . [since he is] an unimpeachable authority who says DNA is too expensive and unnecessary, [and] that NYBC [vaccine is] good."[92]

PATH tried to arrange for both Prince and Maynard to make appearances in Indonesia and Thailand to support Cheil. Success required that PATH carefully orchestrate its allies.

The Different Groups Interested in Fighting Hepatitis B Finally Converge

By early 1986, the three independent streams of activity represented by Maynard, Prince, and Mahoney were coming together, though only on an informal basis. In late January, Shin Seung-il of Eugene Tech/Cheil Sugar proposed that a strategic planning meeting be held, possibly in Seoul, where Maynard would give a public talk. At the meeting representatives of NYBC, CDC, Eugene Tech, PATH, and Cheil could develop a coherent plan. Shin felt that this meeting had to take place before key individuals in Thailand and Indonesia were contacted.[93]

While the group of organizations was moving closer to some formal association, PATH personnel were still investigating whether other vaccines might be superior to the Prince/Cheil vaccine. Wilde, as one of PATH's best-informed advisers, traveled to New York, Paris, and Amsterdam to meet with representatives of three vaccine developers: the NYBC, the Dutch Red Cross, and Pasteur Vaccins.

In his memos to PATH Wilde reported that the plasma-derived hepatitis B vaccines had all been originally developed for the limited purpose of servicing the small market in the developed world. The developers desired a perfect vaccine, one that would receive quick approval by their regulatory authorities. To achieve this goal they chose to utilize high technology and expensive methods to guarantee the highest level of safety. Only after the companies were successful at producing such a hepatitis B vaccine did they realize that the real need was not in the West but in the countries of Asia and Africa. With the exception of the Dutch Red Cross, the major manufacturers were busy working on recombinant DNA vaccines, which were expected to be expensive—"a rich man's product." None of the manufacturers were working on simplifying their vaccine or their production methods to make it appropriate for Indonesia, Thailand, or Africa. If they attempted such work, it would take them years to modify and obtain official approval of the resulting vaccines. This was especially tragic, reported Wilde, because the Merck, Pasteur, and Dutch processes could be easily and safely simplified by just decreasing their use of high technology and/or switching from low-potency to high-potency carrier blood. Wilde concluded his assessment with the comment that the drug companies would continue their policy of charging what the traffic will bear until competition forced them to stop: "people who expect a cheap recombinant [DNA] hepatitis vaccine within the next five years are dreaming."[94] The inescapable conclusion for Wilde was that the Prince/Cheil vaccine was PATH's best bet.

In the spring of 1986, PATH was able to put together a multinational trip to vaccine manufacturers for the Minister of Health of Indonesia. Despite PATH's growing conviction that Cheil was the best vaccine for Asia, it felt obligated to offer the Minister a number of options. Thus, it arranged for the Minister to visit not only NYBC and Cheil but also Merck and KGCC.[95] If the Indonesians decided on their own to work with some company other than Cheil, PATH, despite its own assessment, would lend all the assistance it could to the project.

While dealing with pharmaceutical organizations, PATH discovered that it had to be constantly alert to the aggressive business practices employed by the companies. For instance, when the Minister of Health's party stopped in New York, Mahoney discovered that a key member of the Indonesian group, an important private businessman with close ties to the government, had failed to identify himself as a Merck distributor. This individual aggressively pushed the idea that local production was too risky for Indonesia and suggested that the government should import exclusively from Merck. Mahoney believed that the man successfully worked to keep Mahoney from accompanying the Minister on his planned side trip to Merck headquarters in Pennsylvania.[96] In Seoul, KGCC tried to manipulate the Minister's agenda in a way that would boost its product and discredit Cheil.[97] KGCC officials at the airport managed to get the director of Indonesia's government pharmaceutical company into their car and away from Cheil representatives. Once they had the director in their hands, they raised questions about the quality assurance methods used by the Cheil company and Cheil's use of highly infectious carrier blood. KGCC provoked enough anxiety that the director later made these accusations an issue within the Indonesian government. PATH representatives had to be very quick and vigilant to achieve success in such a high-stakes game.

While in Seoul, Mahoney met with high-ranking Cheil officials as well as with Shin of Eugene Tech. They tried to form a coherent strategy for technology transfer to both Indonesia and Thailand. Both Mahoney and Shin told the Koreans that Cheil was not aggressive enough in marketing the technology-transfer project. The group discussed the importance of setting up two strategies: the first aimed at the distribution of vaccine imported from Korea; the second focused on the establishment of local production facilities. The two approaches would need to be undertaken simultaneously. Cheil and PATH would continue negotiating with an Indonesian private distributor while at the same time working with him to plan for eventual production.[98]

In New York Mahoney had arranged for the Minister of Health of Indonesia to visit the NYBC for a series of discussions, a key one of which was a presentation by Maynard. In his talk, Maynard said that vaccination of high-risk children (those with carrier mothers) would not do enough to lower the high prevalence rates of hepatitis B in developing countries. Rather, "elimination of hepatitis B from human society will require universal immunization [of all children]."[99] Maynard argued that as the demand for the vaccine grew, the price would fall dramatically.

After the Indonesians left, Mahoney stayed behind for a meeting with Maynard, Prince, and Shin.[100] Maynard and Prince aggressively pressed Shin on Cheil's high price and argued for a drop to $1 to $2 a dose.[101] Prince announced that Kenneth Warren, of the Task Force for Child Survival, had stated that UNICEF would not purchase hepatitis B vaccine until it came down to $1 a dose. Any price above that figure constituted the key obstacle to mass immunization campaigns. Maynard also complained that Cheil lacked a person of sufficient experience and stature to lead a high-level international effort effectively.[102] Shin protested that the problem was not lack of commitment by Samsung or Cheil Sugar but rather the lack of effective strategy for promoting hepatitis B vaccination.[103]

The Task Force Is Finally Formed

The group then discussed how a strategy might be developed and who would implement it. Mahoney suggested they adopt an approach similar to that being carried out by the Population Council for the Introduction of Copper T and Norplant contraceptives: form a task force.[104] Maynard, Mahoney, and Prince would be members, but Eugene Tech and Cheil would be excluded, although they would work closely with the new group. It was important, "in order to insure [its] academic status and international credibility, [that] the Task Force should function as an independent, non-commercial entity, sanctioned by NYBC, CDC, WHO and PATH."[105] Mahoney told Shin that financial backing should not come from Cheil. It had to come from philanthropic organizations or the USAID, otherwise the group would lack credibility. Prince emphatically noted that "the task force would not be forever wedded to a Cheil vaccine. . . . [I]f Cheil were not sufficiently responsive to the opportunities the Task Force developed, the Task Force would reserve the right to work with other [vaccine] groups."[106]

Thus, even as Maynard, Prince, and Mahoney coalesced around Cheil Sugar and its vaccine, they put the company on notice that their commitment was not to Cheil but to the goal of mass immunization. If the company did not lend itself to that objective, it would be dispensed with. Cheil would have to understand that message or drop out.

* * *

In summary, in the years before the Task Force was created, a number of individuals and groups were fighting the hepatitis B pandemic in the developing world. They achieved a remarkable degree of success, given their small numbers and their limited resources. Most of them knew each other well and from time to time worked together for specific goals. However, their successes as loosely bound allies or as individuals were severely circumscribed, and their power to affect policy was narrowly restricted. They had the expertise and the commitment but not the means to bring their efforts to fruition. Though individual initiatives and temporary coalitions proved to be insufficient, the groundwork had been laid for a more unified and effective effort in the future. Mahoney, Maynard, and Gust had acquired considerable political sophistication dealing with national and international health politics. They refined their abilities to maneuver through the intricacies of bureaucratic organizations while cultivating important officials. Though Prince was less knowledgeable about health politics, he had a firm grasp of the fundamental problems of vaccine production. These individuals ultimately formed the International Task Force on Hepatitis B Immunization, an entity whose power was greater than the sum of its parts.

Notes

1. According to Prince, as part of their collaboration, he and Blumberg had done research on the physical appearance of the Australian antigen. It looked to Prince remarkably like a virus (though it ultimately turned out to be the surface of a virus, not the virus itself). When he wrote up the material with the title "A New Virus in Human Blood" and asked Blumberg to place his name as co-author, Blumberg refused. In Blumberg's opinion, it was not a virus, but a serum protein that made those who had it susceptible to diseases such as hepatitis. Thus he saw it as associated with hepatitis (and leukemia and leprosy), but not specific to any one of those diseases. After the disagreement, Prince had to develop his own data base, and he discovered what he called the SH antigen, which was specific to hepatitis. The SH antigen and the Australian antigen proved to be identical. Right before Prince published his findings, Blumberg published an article that did in fact identify his antigen with hepatitis. Blumberg, however, despite this major change in direction, was still reluctant to give up his genetic hypothesis, and it kept appearing in his work for some time after his "conversion." Prince says of the situation that as a virologist he was "used to antigens and antibodies," while Blumberg was used

to thinking in terms of genes (Interview with Prince, June 24, 1992). For a good historical overview and relevant references see A. M. Prince, "Detection of Serum Hepatitis Virus Carriers by Testing for the SH (Australia) Antigen: A Review of Current Methodology," *Vox Sanguinus* 19 (1970): 417–424. Also see B. S. Blumberg, W. T. London, A. I. Sutnick, F. R. Camp, Jr., A. J. Luzzio, and N. F. Conte, "Hepatitis Carriers Among Soldiers Who Have Returned from Vietnam: Australia Antigen Studies," *Transfusion* 14 (1974): 63–66; in particular, p. 65, where Blumberg presents an interpretation of his findings that still draws upon his 1967 genetic theory. (For that theory see B. S. Blumberg, B. J. S. Gerstley, D. A. Hungerford, W. T. London, and A. I. Sutnick, "A Serum Antigen [Australia Antigen] in Down's Syndrome, Leukemia and Hepatitis," *Annals of Internal Medicine* 66 [1967]: 924.) Also see the discussion of Prince, Blumberg, and hepatitis B in Allen B. Weisse's excellent study *Medical Odysseys* (New Brunswick, N.J.: Rutgers University Press, 1991), 16–41.

2. Prince says he actually put in a patent for a vaccine before Blumberg did but then withdrew it because it was combined with a diagnostic test that was already outdated.

3. See Alfred Prince, "Prevalence of Serum-Hepatitis-Related Antigen (SH) in Different Geographical Regions," *American Journal of Tropical Medicine and Hygiene* 19 (1970): 872–879.

4. Most of the documents that deal with the International Task Force on Hepatitis B Immunization are found in the files of PATH, the Secretariat organization for the Task Force. I was given unlimited access to those files. I was also given unlimited access to Dr. Prince's files.

5. Interview with Prince, June 24, 1992.

6. Wilde, representing PATH in the period before the Task Force was formed, visited Prince in New York City as part of a fact-finding mission to vaccine manufacturers. After that trip Wilde wrote a memo to his boss that summarized his impression of the international situation (memo from Wilde to Mahoney, Eurasian Trip # 7, January 31, 1986).

7. Interview with Shin, January 24, 1991. (When dealing with Japanese, Korean, and Chinese names I am using the traditional East Asian form of last name first, given name second. In normal English usage, Dr. Shin's name would be written Dr. Seung-il Shin.)

8. It was Shin's belief at the time that the carrier rate was fully 20 percent of the Korean population and that liver cancer was the second most common cancer among men. The actual rate was 8 percent and liver cancer was the third most common cancer (interview with Shin, January 24, 1991).

9. Letter from Prince to Shin, August 6, 1985.

10. He later changed his mind when he realized that WHO's recommendations were both unnecessary and overly biased in favor of the Merck vaccine process.

11. Letter from Prince to Shin, August 6, 1985.

12. Letter from Prince to Shin, October 5, 1985.

13. Letter from Prince to Kenneth S. Warren, M.D., Director of Health Sciences, the Rockefeller Foundation, September 16, 1985.

14. Memo by Mahoney to Hepatitis B File, October 15, 1985, concerning the meeting with Prince.

15. Letter from Prince to Shin, October 2, 1985.

16. Letter from Prince to Shin, June 12, 1986.

17. Interview with Prince, January 29, 1991.

18. Interview with Prince, January 23, 1991.

19. Memo by Mahoney to Hepatitis B File, May 5, 1986, concerning the New York meeting on April 28, 1986, when the Task Force was formed.

20. See the comment by Anthony Robbins and Phyllis Freeman on the politics of health in "Obstacles to Developing Vaccines for the Third World," *Scientific American* (November 1988): 126–133.

21. Interview with Maynard, June 17, 1991.

22. He was originally the head of the CDC's Phoenix "Ecological Investigation Program" in hepatitis. There were two other groups concerned with hepatitis: (1) a surveillance group for hepatitis, which was part of the epidemiological center in Atlanta, Georgia, which did outbreak investigations on request from the individual states; and (2) a laboratory group, which verified serological tests sent them from the various states. Each of the three groups wanted a research component, and thus there were three centers, with a great deal of overlap. By the mid-1970s it became clear that the Phoenix group had achieved primacy over the others. Phoenix had become a WHO Collaborating Centre, and it did the frontline laboratory work on hepatitis. As a result, all hepatitis responsibilities were transferred to it—surveillance, laboratory study, and the Epidemic Intelligence Service office. Ultimately, the Phoenix site was closed down and moved to Atlanta (interview with Maynard, June 17, 1992).

23. Interview with Maynard, June 18, 1992.

24. Interview with Maynard, September 11, 1991.

25. The EPI is a specialized WHO program that "operates primarily as a co-ordinating, advisory and review service for member countries." While it can and does recommend certain vaccines to be used universally, nations themselves decide which vaccines to emphasize and may not adhere to WHO-recommended immunization schedules ("McDonnell Foundation Proposal, A Supplemental Proposal to the James S. McDonnell Foundation to Launch the World's First Immunization Program Against Cancer," December 1986 [in PATH files]).

26. Memo by PATH employee Carl McEvoy to Hepatitis B File, June 19, 1985, concerning the talk with Maynard.

27. As discussed by Mahoney in a memo to Hepatitis B File, November 6, 1985, concerning his first meeting with Maynard.

28. Memo by Carl McEvoy to Hepatitis B File, June 19, 1985.

29. See *WHO Expert Committee on Biological Standardization: Thirty-Fifth Report, Annex 3* (Geneva: World Health Organization, 1983), 70–101.

30. Interview with Maynard, June 17, 1991.

31. While Maynard and others at the CDC's Hepatitis Branch came to believe in the need for universal childhood vaccination in the United States as well, they did not strongly fight for that position during the early to mid-1980s. The Hepatitis Branch people felt that there was almost no support for such a position among their medical and public health constituencies. In addition, no governmental funds were available for such a venture, especially in a period of retrenchment. Instead, they felt compelled to support the existing, ineffectual high-risk strategy that recommended vaccination only for specific targeted groups. They diligently worked to prove the null hypothesis (i.e., to accumulate statistical evidence that the policy did not work). The aggressive and politically sophisticated advocacy of universal childhood vaccination for the

developing world, which would become Maynard's hallmark on the international stage, was not prefigured in his actions on the domestic front: same man, different arenas, different results.

In an interview, Ralph Henderson, head of WHO's EPI, July 1990, told me that many national health leaders find it far easier to work productively on the international level than in their home countries because they are free of domestic restraints and hassles. In an interview I had with Maynard, he denied the validity of Henderson's general observation. I think Maynard's own activities in fact support Henderson's comment. For a complete discussion and critique of American hepatitis B policies, including that of the Hepatitis Branch, CDC, see William Muraskin, "Hepatitis B as a Model (and Anti-Model) for AIDS," in *AIDS and Contemporary History,* edited by Virginia Berridge and Philip Strong (New York: Cambridge University Press, 1993), 108–132; idem, "Individual Rights Versus the Public Health: The Problem of the Asian Hepatitis B Carriers in America," *Social Science and Medicine* 36 (1993): 203–216.

32. Memo by Carl McEvoy to Hepatitis B File, June 1985.

33. Interview with Maynard, June 18, 1991.

34. Ibid.

35. Memo by Carl McEvoy to Hepatitis B File concerning the talk with Maynard, June 19, 1985.

36. Memo by Mahoney to Hepatitis B File concerning the meeting with Maynard, October 2, 1985.

37. Letter from Shin to Prince, September 5, 1985.

38. Memo by Mahoney to Hepatitis B File concerning the first meeting with Maynard, November 6, 1985.

39. Interview with Maynard, June 18, 1991.

40. Interview with Gust, February 24, 1991.

41. Ian Gust, "Toward the Control of Hepatitis B: An Historical Review," *Australian Paediatric Journal* 22 (1988): 273–276.

42. As quoted in *Viral Hepatitis B Infection in the Western Pacific Region: Vaccine and Control,* edited by S. K. Lam, C. L. Lai, and E. K. Yeah (Hong Kong: World Scientific, 1984), 273. One of the other participants also dramatically highlighted the risks of hepatitis B carriership (p. 159): "The risks of HB carriers dying from liver cancers is something like 220 times compared with non-carriers (the risk of smokers getting lung cancer is 10 times only)."

43. In the case of Japanese, Chinese, and Korean names, I am following East Asian custom in giving the individual's surname first and given name second.

44. Ian Gust, "Control of Hepatitis B in the Western Pacific Region," *Medical Journal of Australia* 144 (1986): 473–474, 473.

45. Ibid., 473.

46. Idem, "Toward the Control of Hepatitis B," 121.

47. See John W. Kingdon, *Agendas, Alternatives and Public Policies* (New York: Harper-Collins Publishers, 1984).

48. For a discussion of the politics of WHO, see June Goodfield, *A Chance to Live: The Heroic Story of the Global Campaign to Immunize the World's Children* (New York: Macmillan, 1991), 25–26, where she refers to the WHO regional heads as being similar to feudal barons.

49. There is a persistent myth in the United States, fostered at election time, that foreign aid is a form of disinterested charity. This is not so. When a country helps transfer the technology of one of its companies to another nation it

creates links that later can facilitate other, for-profit business deals. At the least it ties the recipient to future maintenance and supplies from the donor country. In this case the Japanese were the beneficiaries of largesse; other times it has been the Americans, the French, etc.

50. Interview with Gust, February 24, 1991; and interview with Maynard, June 1, 1991.

51. Interview with Maynard, June 1, 1994.

52. Interview with Gust, February 2, 1991.

53. Ibid.

54. Ian Gust, "Public Health Control of HBV: Worldwide HBV Vaccination Programme," in *The Hepatitis Delta Virus,* edited by John L. Gerin, Robert Purcell, and Mario Rizzetto (New York: Wiley-Liss, 1991), 333–342.

55. Interview with Maynard, June 18, 1991.

56. Memo by Mahoney to Hepatitis B File concerning Maynard meeting, March 11, 1986.

57. Interview with Gust, February 24, 1991.

58. Ibid.

59. Interview with Maynard, June 19, 1991.

60. Gust, "Public Health Control of HBV."

61. Ibid.

62. Memo by Mahoney to Hepatitis B File, #13, concerning comments by Beasley to Mahoney, June 26, 1986.

63. PATH is a non-profit organization that was founded in 1980 to "improve health, especially the health of women and children in developing countries." It "focuses on the appropriateness, effectiveness, safety, and availability of technologies for health and family planning." This includes equipment, drugs, devices, vaccines, and procedures used to meet health needs, as well as systems through which health care is delivered. As of 1993 PATH employed 192 people around the world. It has offices in Indonesia, Kenya, Thailand, and the Philippines. It is a WHO Collaborating Centre for Hepatitis B Vaccination, a WHO Collaborating Centre for AIDS, and a WHO Collaborating Centre in Human Reproduction. Since the early 1980s it has received funding to work in 66 developing countries. Between 1987 and 1992 it had revenues of $71,650,000. It has been funded by 80 entities, including institutions and government agencies in 13 countries, 8 multilateral agencies, and 53 foundations and entities. PATH has worked on 115 different specific "technologies" for improving health ("PATH: Facts" [Seattle: PATH, 1993]).

64. Interview with Mahoney, April 29, 1991.

65. Ibid.

66. Memo by Mahoney to Hepatitis B File concerning a conversation with Maynard, October 2, 1985.

67. Interview with Mahoney, April 29, 1991.

68. Ibid.

69. Interview with Mahoney, February 7, 1991.

70. "Hepatitis B Vaccine in Indonesia: An Interim Report to His Excellency Dr. Soewardjono Surjaningrat, The Minister of Health of the Republic of Indonesia" (Seattle: PATH, 1986).

71. Interview with Wilde, April 29, 1991.

72. Ibid.

73. Ibid.

74. Memo by Mahoney to Gordon Perkin, December 13, 1984. This state-

ment of position was in response to a comment from Scott Halstead of the Rockefeller Foundation.

75. Memo of a meeting between Mahoney and Merck officials, April 26, 1985.

76. Ibid.

77. Memo by Mahoney dated October 9, 1985, concerning his conversation with Leona D'Agnes on October 2, 1985.

78. As late as October 9, 1985, Mahoney felt that PATH could work with any of a number of different vaccine manufacturers: the Dutch Red Cross, the Chemo-Sero Therapeutic Institute, the National Institutes of Health, or the NYBC (memo by Mahoney dated October 9, 1985).

79. When Maynard first heard of PATH's desire to transfer technology between private-sector companies, he was skeptical of the "public spiritedness" of such an approach in Thailand. Mahoney spelled out his vision of transferring know-how to the Thai Red Cross with actual production managed by the private sector company. Maynard admitted it was difficult if not impossible for a public sector organization such as the Thai Red Cross to hire and retain qualified people in the highly sophisticated production of modern vaccines, and thus conceded the need for private sector involvement at both ends (memo by Mahoney to Hepatitis B File, August 15, 1985, concerning a talk with Maynard on August 9, 1985).

80. Interview with Mahoney, February 7, 1991.

81. Memo by Mahoney to Hepatitis B File, November 6, 1985.

82. Memo by Mahoney to Hepatitis B File, October 6, 1985, and October 2, 1985.

83. Interview with Mahoney, February 7, 1991.

84. Ibid.

85. Memo by Carl McEvoy to Hepatitis B File, concerning comments after a meeting with Prince on October 9, 1985. While McEvoy's first report to PATH emphasized the NYBC's lack of commercialization skills per se, the problem may have been more specific. As Mahoney put it, "my impression is that the NYBC has been very successful in commercializing inventions made by NYBC staff. What the NYBC had not done was develop a licensing policy that provided for protection of the public sector by . . . requiring that the public sector receive a favorable price," a problem that was to haunt it in its dealing with Cheil (letter from Mahoney to William Muraskin, August 20, 1992).

86. Memo by Mahoney to Hepatitis B File concerning #4 meeting with Prince on October 31, 1985.

87. Anton Widjaya and Leona D'Agnes of PATH-Jakarta had previously prepared "Local Production of Hepatitis B Vaccine, Indonesia: Prefeasibility Study Report" for PATH-Seattle, October 1985.

88. The reasons for this were given in a letter to Dr. Marisi Sihombing, Advisor to the Indonesian Minister of Health, dated October 17, 1985.

89. Memo by Mahoney to Hepatitis B File, December 6, 1985.

90. Ibid.

91. Memo by Mahoney to Hepatitis B File, #5 Seoul Trip, February 18, 1986; letter of February 20, 1986, to Mr. H. K. Kim of Cheil from Mahoney about PATH's work to get distribution agreements in Indonesia and Thailand.

92. Memo by Mahoney to Hepatitis B File, #5 Seoul Trip, February 18, 1986.

93. Memo by Mahoney to Hepatitis B File, January 28, 1986, concerning the meeting with Shin and Prince on January 27–28, 1986.

94. Wilde to Mahoney, Eurasia Trip Report #7, January 31, 1986.

95. Memo by Mahoney to Hepatitis B File, December 6, 1985. Mahoney specifically asked the Minister if he wanted to visit Merck, after the Minister had suggested he visit the NYBC; Mahoney said that he wanted the Minister to continue getting information on his different options.

96. Memo by Mahoney to Hepatitis B File, May 5, 1986, concerning a meeting in New York on April 28, 1986.

97. Memo by Mahoney to Hepatitis B File, May 6, 1985, reporting on activities in Seoul, Korea, from April 23 to 27, 1986.

98. Memo by Mahoney to Hepatitis B File, May 6, 1986.

99. Memo by Mahoney to Hepatitis B File, May 5, 1986.

100. Dr. Kwang Soo Kim, an associate of Shin, was also present.

101. Memo by Mahoney to Hepatitis B File, May 5, 1986.

102. Minutes of the preliminary meeting of the "HB Vaccine Task Force," April 28, 1986, at the NYBC, on a document dated May 2, 1986.

103. Memo by Mahoney to Hepatitis B File, May 5, 1986, reporting on the meeting in New York on April 28, 1986.

104. Memo by Mahoney to Hepatitis B File, May 5, 1986.

105. Maynard was seen as representing both the CDC and WHO in this statement. See the minutes of the preliminary meeting of the "HB Vaccine Task Force," April 28, 1986, at the NYBC, on a document dated May 2, 1986. In a May 5, 1986, memo the Task Force is presented as an NYBC body, with the CDC and PATH helping. In the May 2 statement it is not primarily an NYBC group.

106. Memo by Mahoney to Hepatitis B File, May 5, 1986, giving a summary of the meeting in New York on April 28, 1986.

Chapter 2
The Task Force Takes Shape

The act of creating the International Task Force on Hepatitis B Immunization was more a process than an event, even though one can legitimately point to the specific day (April 28, 1986) the founders agreed to form it. Over time, the group was expanded and reshaped, and it achieved a formal structure that was quite different from the one the founders had originally envisioned. In addition, the new group needed large-scale funding to become more than just another noble but stillborn idea. In this chapter I will look at the Task Force's efforts to find adequate backing and to create links between itself and the powerful organizations that dominated the international health scene. Powerful ideological conflicts raged among those concerned with improving health in the developing world, and the Task Force was forced to pick allies. Certain conditions also persuaded the founders to radically expand the group's membership. In addition, personal contacts and fortunate timing clearly were vital elements in the Task Force's success, without which the dedication, enthusiasm, and expertise of its members would not have been enough.

*   *   *

The formation of the International Task Force on Hepatitis B Immunization radically altered the struggle against hepatitis B and the epidemic of liver cancer that is dependent upon it. The Task Force proved to be far more influential than would have been assumed, given its individual members. While Shin Seung-il, who had been pushing for a strategy meeting for some time, was almost as much the godfather of the Task Force as was Richard Mahoney, the future of the group would be shaped primarily by the latter. For Mahoney the new group was an exciting development because it simultaneously furthered, both for him and for the Program for Appropriate Technology in Health (PATH), vital altruistic and self-interested goals. As he put it in a memorandum, the Task Force "puts PATH on a level with the CDC [Centers for Disease Control], and NYBC [New York Blood Center] in terms of efforts to expand the use of hepatitis B vaccine around the world. It also gives us an opportunity to raise additional funds to support our activities."[1]

Especially attractive for him was the added prestige the group provided for PATH and its programs. When Mahoney spoke to the Indonesian Minister of Health about the new Task Force and the Minister "immediately responded enthusiastically to this plan, indicating that it had the benefit of two nonprofit groups plus the U.S. Government,"[2] Mahoney knew he had achieved the effect he wanted. There existed an initial ambiguity over whether the Task Force was simply made up of individuals who happened to be associated with other organizations or whether the men actually represented those organizations, unofficially or quasi-officially.[3] For Mahoney this was a useful gray area since it allowed outsiders to believe the fledgling group had powerful supporters.[4]

The Task Force Pressures Cheil on Vaccine Price

In the early months of the Task Force in 1986, one of its chief goals was simultaneously to work with and pressure the Cheil Sugar Company regarding the vaccine's pricing. Mahoney, James Maynard, and Alfred Prince relentlessly urged Cheil to establish a $1-a-dose price. They offered that the Task Force would help Cheil establish itself in private sector distribution as a way to recoup the company's investment costs and enable it to offer the vaccine later at $1 a dose to the public sector. Shin doggedly protested that Cheil was "not yet ready to publicly announce"[5] such a low price: first, because it feared it would undercut its effort to make a private sector distribution agreement, and second, because it needed to spell out conditions for the low price (e.g., multivial bottles, large quantities, protection against leakage to the private market, etc.). The Task Force "reaffirmed that [it] . . . is not committed to supporting the Cheil vaccine . . . [but] is committed to assisting in the establishment of national hepatitis immunization programs with a safe and effective vaccine costing less than $1 a dose. If another manufacturer should develop such a vaccine, the Task Force would support it, too."[6]

On a visit to Mahoney in Seattle, H. K. Kim, Managing Director of Cheil, protested that the price could never be set below $1.40–1.50. In addition to problems created by the cost of production, Cheil's competitors (Merck and Pasteur) would be very hostile if Cheil entered the market with a price as low as $1 a dose. Despite these claims Mahoney believed that Cheil's ultimate prosperity was entirely dependent on the success of the Task Force, and that fact gave the Task Force vital leverage. He suggested that Cheil charge whatever it wanted in the private sector and use the profits to make the benchmark $1 a dose possible for the public sector. Kim agreed to report the idea to the heads of the company.[7]

Task Force members also continued to pressure Shin. Because of Shin's status as an academic entrepreneur at Eugene Tech, the mixture of idealism and profit-seeking in his attitude toward the hepatitis B project, in contrast to that of his colleagues at Cheil, was weighted more toward the humanitarian side. Shin firmly believed that the vaccine could not be made for $1 a dose,[8] but he was nevertheless determined to find a way to meet that "uneconomical" price.

Shin first acted as a champion of the $1-a-dose pricing concept when dealing with the leadership of Cheil, but he encountered strong opposition. Cheil was set up to make a profit, and its heads were not in a position to agree to lose money. Cheil had to recover its investment before it could think about a "philanthropic project."[9] Shin boldly decided to go over the heads of Cheil management to the Chairman of the Samsung Conglomerate, Mr. B. C. Lee. Lee's accomplishments made him the Rockefeller and Carnegie of Korea. Certainly within Samsung he had the power to override purely business considerations. The 75-year-old Lee was dying when Shin approached him, and was strongly motivated to make a humanitarian gesture to enhance his reputation.[10] Since hepatitis B was a scourge in Asia, he became convinced that taking decisive action against it would bring honor to his name. (As a consummate businessman he was probably also aware that such a gesture was good public relations for the fledgling Cheil company and its parent, Samsung.) Chairman Lee personally promised to provide compensation for any losses that resulted from selling the vaccine at $1 a dose to the public sector. His guarantee was the major break in the pricing dilemma—one that the Task Force desperately needed.[11] The Task Force could now go to national authorities and international organizations with an affordable vaccine in hand.

While Prince, Maynard, and Mahoney were deeply grateful for Samsung/Cheil's willingness to undercut the outrageously high prices charged elsewhere for the hepatitis vaccine, they were far from convinced that the $1-dose required a completely altruistic mind set. They believed that the low-priced vaccine still offered a profit for Cheil and that other companies could in the future match or beat that offer. (Interestingly, more than six months before Lee offered to subsidize the $1 price, PATH staffer Henry Wilde, with the help of Jonathan Green, an outside U.S. Agency for International Development [USAID] consultant, concluded that hepatitis B vaccine in large quantities would cost no more than six to seven cents to produce. An uncannily accurate forecast, as Mahoney ultimately was to prove.)[12]

The Tie to Cheil Presents Problems and Opportunities

Chairman Lee's offer served to strengthen the already existing links between the Task Force and Cheil. The Cheil vaccine had been the core around which the Task Force had crystallized. But that tie presented significant problems as well as opportunities for the new group. The risks were nowhere better expressed than in the warnings issuing from PATH's representatives in Thailand, Henry Wilde and Donald Douglas. In June 1986 Wilde met with Dr. Supawat Chutivongse, Director of the Thai Red Cross Institute. According to Wilde,

[Dr. Supawat asked] a series of questions . . . intended to clarify whether or not PATH acted as a sales agent for Cheil. He wanted to know whether we had any marketing contracts or other agreements with [Cheil] . . . which would make PATH promote their products. I very emphatically and hopefully correctly assured him that this was not so. . . . This . . . is the third time that I have been grilled on this subject by influential Thai officials.[13]

Wilde and Douglas both believed that the link with Cheil had to be loosened if not broken. They felt the new Task Force should be quickly broadened to include individuals who lacked any ties to Cheil and also clearly possessed connections to other vaccine manufacturers. They went on to argue the importance of the strategy that PATH and the Task Force maintain as much independence as possible:

[C]ompanies, international agencies, and individual countries have such differing agendas that it will be vital for PATH to have a broad network of support to be effective. . . . Most [drug] companies . . . would like nothing more than for the Task Force to go away, because its very existence threaten[s] their profit margins. [They] . . . have the ability to smother an unsupported Task Force. International agencies appear to have other reasons to want this effort to fail, including the widely-accepted priority list of basic, child survival immunization campaigns needed worldwide. . . . [For] national policy reasons, some of the individual countries [sic] efforts [against hepatitis B] . . . may make less than optimum choices. The Task Force should be prepared to work with governments regardless of the nature of the decision taken, and supplier selected. Otherwise, it will not find receptive audiences among government decision makers. . . . If the Task Force were to promote Cheil vaccine exclusively, this will make it a commercial agent . . . in the eyes of intended recipients.[14]

Expansion of the Task Force's Membership

The danger of overidentification of the Task Force with Cheil was strikingly brought home to Maynard as a result of an interaction between Dr. Anton Widjaya, an Indonesian official, and Dr. Fakhry Assaad, Director of the Division of Communicable Diseases, World Health Organization (WHO). During their talk, Widjaya commented that Maynard had done tests that reflected favorably on the potency of the Cheil vaccine. Assaad brushed aside that endorsement and said "Maynard is somewhat biased because [he] . . . might be influenced by his close relationship (frequently 'invited') by that group."[15]

For Maynard, having his independence and status as an authority questioned was intolerable. He had involved himself with the Cheil vaccine because it was the only one that seemed compatible with mass Third World immunization campaigns. This did not involve self-interest: as a senior CDC official he had no right to receive personal remuneration from any drug company for tests, trials, lectures, or other forms of aid he might provide. If monetary benefits were paid they went to the CDC to repay per diem expenses.[16]

The idea that he could be bought by Cheil was as insulting to Maynard as it was dangerous to his reputation. However, Maynard was well aware of the widespread conflicts of interest that plagued the vaccine field. Scientists, with the exception of civil servants like himself, were regularly paid to be on the faculties of drug companies. They also received remuneration for their contributions in trials and tests. As a result, the impartiality of their advice to national and international bodies on the comparative value of different vaccines was often questionable. But Maynard was not going to allow such presumptions to taint his reputation. According to Richard Mahoney, "In reaction to Assaad's comments and based on further thinking and discussion about the Task Force, Maynard came to the conclusion that the Task Force's membership should be expanded, and that it should be more formalized."[17] Mahoney had been thinking along similar lines for some time and had gone so far as to talk with a number of eminent scientists, including R. Palmer Beasley, about joining the Task Force during the months leading up to the Assaad-Widjaya exchange.[18]

In earlier conversations with Wilde, Beasley had shown special interest in the Task Force because he felt that no other group was willing or able to deal with the global problem of fighting hepatitis B. He let Wilde know just how bad he thought the situation actually was:

Dr. Beasley . . . gave us a run down of the attitude of WHO, USAID, and many Ministries of Health toward Hepatitis containment programs. He said that Hepatitis was way down the list of priorities and that the WHO people are still pretty much occupied with the basic EPI [Expanded Programme for Immunization] programs which are eating up more funds than they are able to provide. He feels that one should not count on WHO and USAID when working in this area. . . . A group like [the Task Force] . . . is badly needed since WHO has not paid much attention to this issue, and probably will not in the foreseeable future.[19]

Such views fit in very well with Mahoney's evolving conception of the Task Force. His original idea was not to expand the group itself but to add an advisory council made up of individuals involved in hepatitis research around the world. He mentioned this idea to Maynard as early as July 1986 and found him responsive. Mahoney at that time specifically mentioned Beasley as a possible council member.[20]

In late August and early September 1986 Maynard, Shin, and Prince met in Atlanta and came up with a list of individuals to add directly to the Task Force. Each person was picked on the basis of a particular capacity or background the Task Force lacked. They included:

R. Palmer Beasley, M.D., Professor and Head of the Division of Communicable Disease/Epidemiology, Department of Medicine at the University of California at San Francisco. Beasley was the first to show definitively that hepatitis B was the major cause of liver cancer. His studies were the basis for the current understanding of hepatitis B.

Ian Gust, M.D., Head of the Virus Laboratory at Fairfield Hospital and Director, WHO Laboratory Collaborating Centre for Virus Reference and Research, Melbourne, Australia. Gust had been the principal advisor to the Western Pacific Regional Office (WPRO) of WHO and a member of WPRO's Task Force on Hepatitis B.

Violet How, M.D., Department of Microbiology, University of Malaysia. How had published ground-breaking studies showing that hepatitis vaccine could be included in existing immunization schedules and that hepatitis B vaccine could be given simultaneously with EPI vaccines without harm.

Alain Goudeau, M.D., Institute of Virology, University of Tours. Goudeau was involved in the pioneering efficacy trials for hepatitis B vaccine undertaken in Africa and was the first to show that transmission mechanisms for hepatitis B in Africa were different from those in Asia (i.e., horizontal between children rather than vertical from mother to child).

Xu Xi-Yi, M.D., Chairman and Professor of the Department of Epidemiology of the Shanghai First Medical University. Xu was the first to show that hepatitis B vaccine alone (without the addition of expensive hepatitis B immune globulin) was capable of achieving an efficacy of 90 percent when given to infants of chronic carrier mothers.

E. A. Ayoola, M.D., University of Sokoto, Nigeria. Ayoola had carried out trials showing the practicality of dose reduction in hepatitis B vaccination.

The new members brought both geographic diversity and established relationships with vaccine manufacturers other than Cheil (for example, Goudeau worked on the development of the Pasteur vaccine, and Gust on the Merck vaccine.)[21] Many had had prior relationships with key Task Force founders and had collaborated in earlier efforts to combat the hepatitis B epidemic.

Mahoney felt that giving the Task Force leaders formal titles as officials of the organization would give the group more credibility as an objective source of information. He envisioned Prince as the Chairman, Maynard as the Vice-Chairman, and himself as the Secretary-Treasurer. He also believed it was no longer reasonable for the NYBC to be represented because of its association with Cheil. As part of the Task Force's more formal structure, PATH was asked to become the secretariat for the group, a proposition to which it quickly agreed.[22] In keeping with the desire to separate the Task Force clearly from all vaccine companies, Prince was asked to relinquish his rights to any royalties from the Cheil vaccine. Since his primary goal in developing and nurturing the vaccine was to further mass immunization programs, not make a profit, he readily consented.

Funding from the Rockefeller Foundation

For the new Task Force to be an effective group, large-scale funding was necessary. Initially PATH was able to provide money through one of its grants from USAID—one that supported transfer of health technology to developing countries.[23] However, finding outside funders was vital if the group was to accomplish anything. Mahoney had worked for the Ford Foundation for a number of years and had contacts in that organization, but he knew that a long-standing agreement existed between the Ford and the Rockefeller Foundations specifying that the latter would handle health matters. Mahoney was aware that Dr. Kenneth Warren, Director of Health Sciences at Rockefeller, would be an important contact for the Task Force, but he did not know him personally. Mahoney arranged to meet with Warren and decided to bring Dr. Gordon Perkin, the President of PATH, with him, believing that Perkin's stature and prestige in the health field would give Mahoney's presentation added weight.

Unbeknownst to Mahoney, Perkin's presence offered a far better entrée to Warren than did his good reputation in the health community. Perkin previously had been instrumental in furthering a project of personal significance to Warren, who, after he obtained his medical degree, had been very interested in tropical medicine and by the problem of schistosomiasis—the most important parasitic liver disease in the world. Warren developed a simple and inexpensive test for the disease, and Perkin, working through PATH, had helped arrange to have it mass produced.[24]

Thus Warren was favorably disposed to Perkin (and PATH) because of his past experience with them, and his work in hepatology with schistosomiasis made him keenly aware of the significance of the hepatitis B problem. It was his belief that simultaneous infection with schistosomiasis and hepatitis B, a not uncommon situation, exaggerated the effects of both diseases. Indeed, previously he had done experiments on mice at the National Institutes of Health that focused directly on the implications of dual infections of the liver.[25]

As a result, Warren was enthusiastic about the idea of a hepatitis B task force. Fortunately, the rules of the Rockefeller Foundation made it possible for him to translate his excitement directly into practical support. As Director of Health Sciences, Warren had the power on his own initiative, without consultation, to grant up to $50,000 to a worthwhile project. He could thus avoid the normal delays of formal application and review procedures. Using that power he proceeded to give the Task Force $50,000 as seed money until a larger grant could be obtained.[26]

To some extent Mahoney's seeking out of Warren at Rockefeller had been forced on him by the failure to produce results via his more intimate links to people at the Ford Foundation. Being shifted over to Rockefeller, however, turned out to be exceptionally fortunate because Warren was more than a gatekeeper for seed money, he was a key player in the global movement for universal vaccinations in the Third World.

Warren and the Debate over International Vaccination Programs

In 1979, Kenneth Warren and Julia Walsh had written a seminal article on a strategy for disease control in developing countries.[27] The article was an interim alternative to, and implicit critique of, the policy adopted by WHO in 1978 which called for comprehensive primary health care as the solution to death and disability in the developing world. According to WHO's "Declaration of Alma-Ata,"[28]

Primary health care . . . includes at least: education concerning prevailing health problems . . . promotion of food supply and proper nutrition; an adequate supply of safe water and basic sanitation; maternal and child health care . . . immunization against the major infectious diseases . . . [and] requires and promotes maximum community and individual self-reliance and participation in the planning, organization, operation and control of primary health care.[29]

For Warren and Walsh, "The goal set at Alma Ata is above reproach, yet its very scope makes it unattainable. . . . It would cost billions of dollars to provide minimal, basic (not comprehensive) health services"[30] to the world's poor. The cost of clean water and sanitation alone would be astronomical. The World Bank estimated the cost of providing community water and sanitation at 135 to 260 billion dollars, and this excluded the cost of hookups to individual houses, which would be required to achieve maximum health benefits.[31]

In addition, the Alma Ata declaration envisioned fundamental economic, social, and political transformation as indispensable to the provision of adequate health care:

Health . . . is a state of complete physical, mental and social well-being, and not merely the absence of disease or infirmity. . . . [T]he people have the right and duty to participate individually and collectively in the planning and implementation of their health care. . . . Economic and social development, based on a New International Economic Order, is of basic importance to the fullest attainment of health . . . and the reduction of the gap between the health status of the developing and developed countries.[32]

Because none of these political/economic transformations had a high probability of occurring in the near future, Warren and Walsh, while waiting for the conditions necessary for comprehensive primary health care to come into existence, called for a policy of selective primary health care in which a small group of health problems would be chosen (on the basis of their contribution to total mortality, the availability of a cheap and effective cure or preventative, and their overall cost/benefit ratio) and intensively combated.

This type of policy, called the vertical approach, utilizes "direct, targeted programs, using specific technologies such as drugs, vaccines, and insecticides,"[33] in contrast to the comprehensive primary health care, or horizontal approach, "which simultaneously utilize[s] all means—medical, ecological, sociological, and political—to improve health."[34]

Rivalry between vertical and horizontal programs can be traced back in public health circles for more than 100 years. Recently, the dramatic failure of certain high-profile vertical campaigns, especially the failure of the anti-malaria crusade, created "a major backlash, not only against the strategy of disease eradication but against the vertical approach in general."[35] As a result the horizontal approach became more attractive, and many observers, according to Warren, saw general "socioeconomic development as a panacea for all the less developed world's ills."[36]

This anti-vertical view was provided significant support by the writings of the medical historian Thomas McKeown. His work has argued that the source of improving health in the developed world in the nineteenth and twentieth centuries has come not from medical interventions but rather from the rising standard of living, especially improvements in nutrition. Neither immunization nor clinical medical treatment has been particularly helpful or useful. His views have become dominant in key intellectual circles in the West and have lent themselves to the anti-medicine and anti-technology backlash that has grown in recent years.[37]

In Warren and Walsh's eyes, by the time of the Alma Ata conference "primary health care within a decidedly horizontal framework had become a crusade . . . [and] other approaches to improve health in the less developed world were often treated as heresies."[38] Nevertheless, in their article they recommended vertical campaigns utilizing immunization against tuberculosis, polio, measles, diphtheria, whooping cough, and tetanus; use of oral rehydration therapy against diarrheal diseases; treatment for malaria; and breast-feeding of infants.[39]

Mahoney knew that hepatitis B vaccination as a vertical campaign would fit well with Warren's support of selective primary health care since it met all of the necessary conditions: hepatitis B had (long-term) high mortality, there was an effective and potentially inexpensive preventative, and there was a good cost/benefit ratio in immunizing against it. Neither Mahoney nor the Task Force had a strong theoretical position in favor of vertical programs or against horizontal ones; instead, it was simply a practical matter—they had a vaccine, and their expertise revolved around perfecting it and delivering it. They did not have the competence nor the tools to effect general social-economic-political change.[40]

To the extent that Task Force members thought about the strident controversy agitating public health officials, they saw the problem less as a struggle over fundamental principles than as a bureaucratic turf fight. WHO held the United Nations mandate to deal with global health and was doing so by championing a pro-horizontal health strategy as promulgated by the Declaration of Alma Ata. UNICEF (United

Nations Children's Fund) had only recently decided to enter the health field and had adopted a Warrenesque program it called the Child Survival Revolution. Its strategy was "based on widespread adoption of a small number of cheap, accessible and simple technologies,"[41] referred to by the acronym GOBI (growth monitoring, oral rehydration therapy, breast feeding, and immunization).[42] UNICEF's initial efforts focused primarily on immunization.[43]

Task Force members believed that UNICEF's initiative on health issues was a direct threat to WHO's prerogatives and prestige as the leader in health matters. Other issues in the debate either seemed of secondary importance or were ignored by the Task Force, for which the relevant question was always the practical one (i.e., What will combat the hepatitis B epidemic most quickly, cheaply, and effectively?). They could not wait for the best of all possible worlds; they could only work for a better one right now.[44]

For many radical health planners and intellectuals such an outlook is a hallmark of capitalistic thinking that hides its conservative bias under the false claim of being non-ideological.[45] For them, vertical programs, or selective primary health care, are nothing short of counterrevolutionary activity.[46] For such critics the horizontal approach of Alma Ata was the opening shot in a revolutionary transformation of Third World society. As one commentator put it:

[Alma Ata's emphasis on community self-reliance and social control over medical technology] mark[ed] a watershed and probably the most important one in the history of medicine and public health. . . . UNICEF [by its policies] and its powerful backers are in fact contributing to reverse this historic gain of the people . . . by making people once again dependent on Western countries for funds, vaccines, and equipment. . . . There is an ominous similarity between the spread of a highly malignant tumor and the promotion of the technocratic approach by Western countries. . . . Vested interests have struck back by glorifying the work of Walsh and Warren.[47]

Or as a more moderate observer put it:

PHC [primary health care] was crystallized as an approach at a time when there was wide agreement that the causes of poverty were nonnatural and that social justice was a requisite for health. . . . UNICEF [post–Alma Ata policy] locates health action wholly outside the realm of socioeconomic rights and responsibilities. . . . [A] hundred . . . "appropriate technologies" have become a substitute for social transformation. . . . The "Children's revolution" is a minimal package in the face of the failure of parents to achieve a revolution in the power relations determining health.[48]

For such critics, groups like the International Task Force on Hepatitis B Immunization are little better than a form of reactionary paternalism since such vertical programs create their "limited package of interventions outside of the local situation. . . . [and reduce the populations' input to an] acceptance of the package, as recipients of the 'message' but not as transformers of their own situation."[49] Such programs undermine any challenge to repressive governmental structures because the vertical programs depend upon entrenched elite aid, and thus "in both symbolic and practical ways the power of national structures of dominance are reinforced in these campaigns."[50]

As a result of their philosophical position, many of these observers believe that even if vertical campaigns such as hepatitis B immunization worked, they would still be less than useless because if such programs

are [effectively] applied to a total population, the health system may still be classed as a failure. If what results is still an oppression, does not deal with that society's priorities . . . then it is not successful. [In addition] . . . a PHC [primary health care] system can still be classed as successful even if some of the illnesses and deaths targeted by . . . [vertical programs] continue to occur *if* that society truly has a choice but decides to take up other priorities knowing the implications.[51]

For Mahoney, Maynard, and Prince such an uncompromising position, which sees failure in success and success in failure (the dead and dying notwithstanding), was grotesque and unconscionable. They did not oppose major social change or empowerment of the local people, but saw that such goals could not justify allowing needless death and morbidity to continue unchecked. In fighting disease one uses the resources at hand, even if some of the resources are not those one would freely choose.

The radical critics' dismissal of vertical programs because the technologies are used by ruling elites "to achieve visible . . . improvements in health to divert attention away from the lack of basic survival needs"[52] makes little sense, as dramatic improvements in health are of fundamental importance to human beings regardless of diversionary side effects. Better health is a real benefit to the recipient, while the label diversionary is at best an interpretation, and a rather elitist one, since it replaces the actual view of a population with what the critic claims the people should feel.

Mahoney and the Task Force for Child Survival

Thus, for the International Task Force on Hepatitis B Immunization, Warren and his interim strategy for active disease fighting were both appealing and convincing in a way his left-wing critics were not. Warren represented a potential supporter and immediate source of much-

needed funds, and in addition he offered access to a major international power center: the prestigious Task Force for Child Survival.

The Task Force for Child Survival was an organization whose membership was composed of representatives from several major institutions. The original convening members were UNICEF, WHO,
the Rockefeller Foundation, the United Nations Development Programme, and the World Bank. The idea for it had come out of a series
of meetings between Jonas Salk and Robert MacNamara. As Warren
remembered the situation:

> It was Salk's contention that . . . [the] Expanded Programme on Immunization,
> [the World Health Organization's major concession to vertical campaigns] . . .
> was moving too slowly. Salk and MacNamara had been working on develop-
> ment of an independent agency to spearhead the immunization effort, but
> after hearing of UNICEF's children's revolution they came to try to convince
> [Jim] Grant [head of UNICEF] to take over the leadership. . . . To that end, a
> meeting was organized . . . and [an] ad hoc Task Force for Child Survival was
> formed to develop both country programs and research aspects of accelerated
> immunization activities.[53]

(Though Warren modestly leaves his own pivotal role in the creation of
the Task Force for Child Survival out of this account, he elsewhere
stated, "I organized the Task Force in 1984."[54] Warren felt that the new
hepatitis B Task Force was modeled on his Task Force for Child Survival, and that belief increased its attractiveness to him.)[55]

At least initially, the Child Survival group appeared to Mahoney to
be the coordinating center for the world's immunization activities and
to have the power, prestige, and money that the new Task Force on
hepatitis B needed to be effective. (Later, he came to feel that the group
was less important because it did not directly involve itself in initiating
projects but primarily served as a facilitator for its constituent organizations to meet and discuss problems.) At this point its help appeared
to be vitally necessary for the new hepatitis B group.

The first thing Warren did was to invite Mahoney to give a presentation to the Task Force for Child Survival at its next meeting. Mahoney
saw the invitation as a major opportunity for the fledgling hepatitis B
Task Force[56] because it offered the possibility of obtaining funding and
because it bettered the odds for having Maynard join the prestigious
group. What a coup that would be![57]

The mere fact that Mahoney was invited to speak to the Task Force
for Child Survival significantly helped establish the new organization's
credentials. It automatically made the Task Force on hepatitis B very
marketable, regardless of the level of concrete aid the child-oriented
group would provide.[58] Later, when Mahoney corresponded with the
Minister of Health of Indonesia and discussed the formation of the

hepatitis B Task Force, he highlighted the invitation and carefully emphasized the organizations that composed it as a means of achieving prestige by association for his group.[59]

The discussion that took place during the meeting was considerably more ambiguous. Newton Bowles, personal advisor to James Grant of UNICEF, was not supportive at all. He expressed a layman's skepticism about the importance of hepatitis B, especially as a child survival issue. He said that other vaccines, such as those for malaria, cholera, and rotavirus, would come along in the near future and that the Task Force for Child Survival should give them higher priority. UNICEF, said Bowles, would only be a vital player if universal vaccination for hepatitis B ever become a reality.[60] As one observer archly commented, Bowles came from UNICEF, and "all he cared about was children; he did not care about those who die at 50."[61]

It was gratifying for Mahoney that Warren, William Foege (ex-Director of the CDC and Chairman of the Task Force for Child Survival), and Ralph Henderson, head of WHO's EPI, vigorously opposed Bowles's view by pointing out that hepatitis B was clearly an important problem for children since they became infected during childhood. Foege went on to argue that Bowles himself, as a China expert, should be deeply concerned that three-fourths of the infected people in the world were Chinese. Nevertheless, it was quite disappointing when Henderson of EPI firmly stated that WHO/UNICEF funding was totally committed to the present six universal vaccines (tuberculosis, diphtheria, pertussis, tetanus, polio, and measles) and had nothing left for hepatitis B. To make matters worse, Henderson was strongly opposed to the idea of local vaccine production in Indonesia, something the International Task Force was enthusiastic about. He pointedly stressed his hope that they would actively discourage the Indonesians. Such views were not what Mahoney needed to hear.

The lack of an offer of financial aid to the new Task Force was to some extent offset by "the general theme of the conversation . . . that hepatitis B because of its association with liver cancer would be politically attractive to [the] bilateral donors [who would see it as] . . . The War on Cancer."[62] Another positive development was that Foege asked how the Task Force for Child Survival could help, and Henderson expressed his general support for the new undertaking, despite his stated reservations.[63] Most important of all, the invitation had been a goodwill gesture on Warren's part, constituting an attempt to give the new Task Force exposure and proving his willingness to put his international reputation on the line for it.[64]

Nevertheless, the meeting highlighted a problem that the hepatitis B Task Force would face for years to come: private donors, international organizations, and national governments were all oriented toward helping children. The image of suffering children is a powerful one. The fact that children's lives depend upon the ability of their middle-aged fathers and mothers to earn a living may make intellectual sense but has less emotional impact. As a result, the Task Force found itself forced to present hepatitis B as an issue of child survival.

The McDonnell Foundation

Far more important than the seed money Warren supplied or the invitation to the Task Force for Child Survival meeting that he extended was his role in finding large-scale financing for the hepatitis B Task Force. It is because of Warren's efforts in this area that Mahoney attributes to him the key role in making the Task Force a reality. At his first meeting with Mahoney, Warren said, rather cryptically, that he knew of someone who might be interested in supporting their efforts. He would not tell Mahoney who it was, probably because this individual was still in the process of competing for the job of foundation president and had not yet obtained it.[65]

The man was John Bruer, Ph.D. Bruer was a Warren protégé who had worked under him for a few years at the Rockefeller Foundation. When headhunters came looking for a president for the James S. McDonnell Foundation, Warren strongly recommended Bruer.[66] Even before Bruer had been interviewed by the McDonnell board, Warren spoke to him about the hepatitis B Task Force. Warren pointed out that the hepatitis B vaccine could be seen as the first anti-cancer vaccine since primary liver cancer was overwhelmingly correlated with a previous hepatitis B virus infection. During Bruer's Foundation interview, it became clear that the McDonnell family had a personal interest in cancer prevention, and James McDonnell III actually asked Bruer what he would do to support the fight against cancer. Bruer told him that throwing money into cancer research was easy but not of great significance, especially for a small foundation. However, there was an International Task Force on Hepatitis B Immunization that was planning to conduct field tests on the feasibility of mass vaccination campaigns. This work, if supported, might represent a significant contribution by the Foundation.[67]

Bruer was ultimately chosen as the President of the McDonnell Foundation. Soon afterward, Warren gave the hepatitis B Task Force Bruer's name and suggested that it contact him. It did so. Prince, Mahoney, Maynard, and a member of his CDC staff, Dr. Mark Kane, went to St. Louis in November 1986 to make their presentation. Their subsequent proposal was submitted to the board and approved. In the end the Foundation funded the Task Force for three years, with a grant of almost two and a half million dollars.[68] Support by the McDonnell Foundation changed the Task Force from a noble idea into a functioning organization.[69]

Bruer and the McDonnell Foundation thus became the instruments for launching the hepatitis initiative. Bruer's knowledge of the existence of the new organization may indeed have been instrumental in his being appointed President of the Foundation. The grant the McDonnell Foundation gave the Task Force in turn constituted "a step toward establishing [the Foundation's] visibility in the international arena"[70] and helped it begin a major transformation from a local institution into an international player. Thus Bruer and the McDonnell Foundation helped make the Task Force, and the Task Force helped make the Foundation and Bruer, while Warren and the Rockefeller Foundation acted as godfathers during the whole process.[71]

The Proposal to the McDonnell Foundation

The Task Force's grant proposal, entitled "A Proposal to Launch the First International Immunization Program Against Hepatitis B and Primary Cancer of the Liver," was a very ambitious and sweeping one. Submitted to the McDonnell Foundation in November 1986, it began by declaring that:

Hepatitis B Virus (HBV) is second only to tobacco as a cause of cancer. It leads to the development of liver cancer and in developing countries this cancer strikes down primarily men in their most productive years. . . . Hepatitis B virus is highly endemic . . . with prevalences of infection reaching 95% in most parts of sub-Saharan Africa and Southeast Asia. The infection results in chronic virus carriage in between 5% and 30%. . . . These chronic carriers provide a pool for further infection . . . [and there are] almost 300 million worldwide.[72]

It set out two key objectives:

1. Determine practical means for integrating hepatitis B immunization into programs for mass immunization of infants.
2. Stimulate the production of hepatitis B vaccines in sufficient quantities and at low prices to enable developing countries to undertake programs of mass infant immunization.[73]

The proposal also laid out a series of impressive measurable objectives:

1. Undertake demonstration projects in four countries involving the immunization of over 1 million children.

2. Complete a program of information dissemination to all developing countries where hepatitis B is hyper-endemic to heighten awareness and commitment on the part of the national health authorities. . . .
3. Help to establish local production of hepatitis B vaccine in at least two countries in hyper-endemic regions.
4. Provide the basis for integration of hepatitis B vaccination into the Expanded Programme on Immunization [EPI] of WHO.[74]

The Task Force announced that the basis for the selection of the countries for demonstration projects would be the existence of political will (as affirmed at the highest governmental level) and resources to put in place a nationwide immunization program once its feasibility had been shown. The overall objective, however, would be to show that hepatitis B could be added to the WHO's EPI.[75]

The demonstration projects would also be used to study important practical questions that could affect future immunization programs: the possibility of going beyond the cold chain (i.e., beyond the need to keep the vaccines constantly cold, which raised the cost and lowered the effectiveness of mass vaccination campaigns); the usefulness of multivalent vaccines (i.e., the combining of different vaccines such as diphtheria-pertussis-tetanus and hepatitis B into one shot); and the amount of latitude in the timing of the shots.[76]

Second in importance to the demonstration projects only was the goal of aiding in the local production of hepatitis B vaccine. Only a few developing countries would be candidates for such a venture—those with approximately fifty million people, a good technical infrastructure, the political motivation to support local production, and the willingness to make long-term financial commitments. Key candidates would be Indonesia, Thailand, Brazil, Egypt, India, Pakistan, and Turkey.

The country chosen for the first demonstration project was Indonesia. The Task Force had already held meetings with the Indonesian Minister of Health, who requested that it submit a plan for launching a national immunization project. PATH, the Task Force's secretariat, had already spent a year working to assist in the establishment of local hepatitis B vaccine production. Four private pharmaceutical companies were interested in setting up production of vaccines (Cheil, Korean Green Cross Corporation, Merck Sharp & Dohme, and Pasteur Vaccins). Each would work through a local joint venture partner. Once the government decided on the vaccine it wanted, the Task Force would help provide technical assistance such as arranging training of production staff, developing a national quality assurance capability for hepatitis B vaccines at the Ministry of Health Laboratories, and establishing regulations for the control of production by the government. The Task Force would work closely with private industry.[77]

The Task Force informed the McDonnell Foundation that the commitment of one manufacturer (Cheil) had provided the reason for the group to form in the first place. However, this did "not represent a commitment on the part of the Task Force to endorse, support, or use the vaccine of the committing manufacturer."[78]

The Task Force pointed out that the part of the program that was most likely to meet with major delays was the transfer of vaccine production technology:

The major reason for delay is the large number of independent centers that participate in technology transfer projects. . . . [I]n Indonesia the power centers are: the Ministry of Health, the Ministry of Industry, the Ministry of Science and Technology, the Food and Drug Administration, the local company, the source of technology, competitors of the technology source, WHO, banks to finance the project, bilateral donor agencies, et al.[79]

In later years, though the Task Force would receive significant aid from many sources, the McDonnell Foundation would remain a key supporter. At the end of the three years, the grant was renewed for another two million dollars. President Bruer was very impressed with the quality of the men and women who ran the Task Force and its operations. He was especially pleased by the fact that they possessed "real compassion for people,"[80] and he was excited by the fact that they were "Indiana Joneses with brains."[81] He also appreciated the ethnic/national diversity of the expanded Task Force, with dedicated experts from Asia, Europe, Africa, and the Middle East. He found its meetings, unlike most group discussions, highly democratic and egalitarian.[82] (In turn, the Task Force was impressed by Bruer's ability to observe heated, emotional debates without losing sight of the unity and collegial bonds that made unpleasant truth-telling possible.[83] The normal processes of "group think" that make for an artificial consensus in organizations was not allowed to operate in the Task Force.)

*   *   *

In sum, what has become clear in this chapter is that the decision to create the hepatitis B Task Force could only become meaningful if a significant source of funding could be found. The Rockefeller Foundation, as personified by Warren, was the key to the Task Force founders' successful search. Warren supplied the seed money to allow the Task Force to function and to provide time for the group to seek more

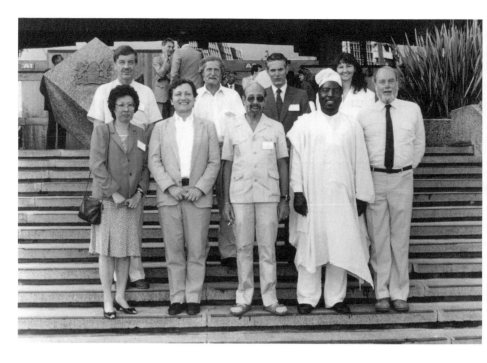

Nairobi Task Force meeting, March 1987. *Left to right, back row:* Dr. James Maynard, Dr. Ian Gust, Dr. Richard Mahoney, Nancy Muller; *front row:* Dr. Violet How, Dr. Alain Goudeau, Dr. Alfred Prince, Dr. E. A. Ayoola, Dr. R. Palmer Beasley.

support. In addition, his money was used to sponsor a donors' meeting in New York City, where the Task Force was introduced to potential funders. It was also used to finance the Task Force's first annual meeting in March 1987, in Nairobi, Kenya, where the individuals who made up the expanded membership met each other for the first time and formally constituted the new group. It was at this conference that the group was able to meet representatives of the major international pharmaceutical companies and declare its desire for a low-cost vaccine, priced to allow mass immunization campaigns.[84]

As we have seen, even more important than providing the seed money, Warren helped the Task Force get major funding by bringing the group together with John Bruer of the McDonnell Foundation. Without the personal and professional connection between Warren and Bruer, neither Bruer nor the Task Force would have known of the other's existence, let alone become collaborators.

We have also seen that there was a major division among public health experts about the role of immunization programs in the developing world. Many people who attacked vaccination programs spoke of them as little more than Western technological imperialism. Despite the strong socialist leanings of many of the Task Force founders, this jaundiced view was almost incomprehensible to them. On this key point they found themselves firmly allied with those groups that favored the aggressive use of vaccines to prevent disease.

Once the Task Force was fully funded and organized, its next step was to set up model projects in the developing world to prove that mass immunization was both affordable and practical. In the following chapter we will look at the first such program, which was established in the Republic of Indonesia.

Notes

1. Memo by Mahoney to Hepatitis B File, May 5, 1986, concerning the meeting in New York on April 28, 1986.
2. Ibid.
3. As late as July 21, 1986, Henry Wilde could write to an important Thai academic that "PATH, Cheil, New York Blood Center and the Dutch Red Cross are forming a Task Force" (letter from Wilde to Prof. Dr. Prasert Thongcharoen, Chairman, Department of Microbiology, Sirirja Hospital Faculty of Medicine).
4. In an interview Mahoney said that the Task Force was always composed of individuals and never represented organizations per se. Some early documents support that position, others do not. In a June 4, 1986, memo (#1) from Mahoney, reporting on a May 29–30, 1986, meeting, he talks about "the Task Force (i.e. PATH, NYBC, CDC) organizing . . . [a] meeting." The fact that the Task Force for Child Survival, which was made up of representatives from WHO, UNICEF, the World Bank, and the United Nations Development Programme, was initially seen as a model for the International Task Force on Hepatitis B Immunization may have led to this early emphasis.
5. Memo by Mahoney to Hepatitis B File, June 4, 1986, East Coast Trip #1, concerning the meeting in New York May 23–30, 1986.
6. Ibid.
7. Memo by Mahoney to Hepatitis B File, May 14, 1986.
8. Interview with Shin, January 24, 1991.
9. Letter from Shin to Maynard, June 2, 1986.
10. Interview with Shin, January 24, 1991.
11. Letter from Shin to Members of the Task Force, August 15, 1986.
12. Jonathan A. Green, "Report to PATH Re Health Link Project: Subproject Review January and February 1986," addressed to USAID, which required the review of its grantee, PATH. See Richard Mahoney, "The Cost of EPI Vaccine Production with Special Reference to Hepatitis B Vaccine" (PATH files). Of course such low figures (six to seven cents a dose) did not include retrieving the original costs of developing the vaccine or its cost when produced in relatively small amounts. Great savings occur, as in any manufacturing process, when large quantities are produced, and the price falls to little

more than the cost of raw materials. Prince's concept of $1 a dose, needless to say, was obtainable at much lower levels of production. However, he assumed that the European/American companies, with their higher developmental and production costs, could meet the $1-a-dose price by charging higher prices to the private sector—especially in the developed world. The drug companies have long claimed that they could afford to provide the six universal Expanded Programme for Immunization vaccines at very low prices only because they subsidized them with profits from the private market. Until recently Prince accepted that argument and the necessity for a dual market and pricing policy (i.e., high vaccine prices in the industrial world so that public sector prices could be low in the developing world). Many in the United States, including representatives in Congress, do not accept the legitimacy of this two-tier system, and Prince himself seems to have developed doubts about its continued necessity. Lacking access to the cost records of the European/American companies makes it impossible to say how high a one-tier price for vaccines would have to be to retrieve developmental costs and provide a reasonable return on capital. Task Force strategy, however, has been based on accepting the companies' strategy of charging what the traffic will bear in the private sector to obtain low public sector prices.

13. Memo by Wilde to Hepatitis B File, dated June 8, 1986. The meeting appears to have been a luncheon with Supawat. The memo has Wilde's signature but it could have been written by Douglas of PATH-Thailand.

14. Memo by Wilde and Douglas to Hepatitis B File, June 15, 1986, concerning comments on the Task Force on Hepatitis B/nominations for membership on the Task Force.

15. Memo by Widjaya to Leona D'Agnes, PATH-Jakarta.

16. Interview with Maynard, June 19, 1991.

17. Memo by Mahoney to Gordon W. Perkin, President of PATH, September 4, 1986.

18. At an international conference sponsored by Pasteur Vaccins, Mahoney suggested consideration be given to forming a subgroup of individuals, from among those attending, to undertake efforts to get hepatitis B immunization in developing countries a higher priority. Both Dr. Beasley and Dr. Violet How (both of whom later joined the Task Force) said they were interested in working with PATH on such a venture. Beasley said he liked the Task Force that PATH was attempting to organize, and he and How recommended several individuals who should be invited (memo by Mahoney to Hepatitis B File, #13, June 26, 1986).

19. Memo by Wilde to Hepatitis B File, June 14, 1986, concerning breakfast with Dr. Beasley et al.

20. Memo by Mahoney to Hepatitis B File, July 7, 1986, regarding a telephone conversation with Maynard on July 7.

21. Memo by Mahoney to Gordon W. Perkin, President of PATH, September 4, 1986; letter from Mahoney to Dr. S. Soewardjono, Minister of Health of Indonesia, September 5, 1986; and letter from Mahoney to Soewardjono, dated September 25, 1986.

22. Memo by Mahoney to Gordon W. Perkin, September 4, 1986. At the beginning Mahoney envisioned the Task Force as an activity of the NYBC. Later he believed that the more formalized Task Force would be seen as an activity of PATH. This view was not shared by the other Task Force members, and later it would become a significant cause of conflict within the group.

23. Letter from Mahoney to Dr. Ralph Henderson, head of the WHO's EPI, dated October 6, 1986.

24. Interview with Warren, November 18, 1991.

25. Ibid.

26. Ibid.

27. Kenneth Warren and Julia Walsh, "Selective Primary Health Care: An Interim Strategy for Disease Control in Developing Countries," *New England Journal of Medicine* 301 (1979): 967–974. For the first time mortality and morbidity data were separated in developing countries to highlight the specific diseases that were killing children. This simple disaggregating procedure (which, though obvious, had not been done before) made it clear that millions of child deaths were occurring annually from a few diseases that were avoidable by inexpensive and easily manageable interventions.

28. WHO called the meeting, but the Declaration was supported by many organizations, including UNICEF.

29. See Kenneth S. Warren, "The Alma-Ata Declaration: Health for All by the Year 2000?" in *Encyclopedia Britannica, 1990 Year Book,* 22.

30. Warren and Walsh, "Selective Primary Health Care."

31. Ibid.

32. Warren, "The Alma-Ata Declaration," 22.

33. Ibid., 25.

34. Ibid.

35. Ibid.

36. Ibid.

37. Ibid. See, for example, Thomas McKeown, *The Role of Medicine: Dream, Mirage, or Nemesis* (Princeton, N.J.: Princeton University Press, 1979). One of the few historians to try aggressively to refute McKeown by original research has been Leonard G. Wilson; see Leonard G. Wilson, "The Historical Decline of Tuberculosis in Europe and America: Its Causes and Significance," *Journal of History of Medicine and Allied Sciences* 45 (1990): 366–396; idem, "The Rise and Fall of Tuberculosis in Minnesota: The Role of Infection," *Bulletin of the History of Medicine* 66 (1992): 16–52. But even these two works are more modifications of McKeown's thesis than actual refutations since they implicitly accept much of McKeown's debunking of the claims of medicine's pivotal role. An even more sweeping attack on the McKeown thesis can be found in Simon Szreter, "The Importance of Social Intervention in Britain's Mortality Decline, c. 1850–1914: A Reinterpretation of the Role of Public Health," *Social History* 1 (1988): 1–37. Also see Anne Hardy, *The Epidemic Streets: Infectious Disease and the Rise of Preventive Medicine, 1856–1900* (Oxford: Clarendon Press, 1993).

38. Warren, "The Alma-Ata Declaration," 26.

39. Ibid., 27.

40. Interview with Mahoney, December 2, 1991.

41. Benjamin Wiener, "GOBI versus PHC? Some Dangers of Selective Primary Health Care," *Social Science and Medicine* 26 (1988): 963–969.

42. Later GOBI was expanded to GOBI-FFF (family spacing, female literacy, and feeding).

43. Warren, "The Alma-Ata Declaration," 27.

44. For example, soon after the formation of the Task Force, Maynard and Prince put together a fragile alliance involving the Brazilian government, the Oswaldo Cruz Institute, and the Japanese Aid Organization to make producing an inexpensive hepatitis B vaccine in Brazil possible as the first step toward

a mass immunization program. That potentially fruitful alignment collapsed, at least according to some members of the Task Force, when an impractical but more idealistic approach was championed by a prestigious outside expert (interview with Maynard, June 18, 1991).

45. See Vicente Navarro, "A Critique of the Ideological and Political Position of the Brandt Report and the Alma Ata Declaration," *International Journal of Health Services* 14 (1984): 159–173. Navarro suggests "Individuals may be unconscious bearers of ideologies and practices that serve quite different purposes from the ones individually and consciously desired." For example, he talks of the Pan-American Health Organization as showing its class bias by "a consistent presentation of empirical and functionalist positions, i.e. the dominant ideologies in Western academic circles," views that are made to appear apolitical when they are actually very political (164–165). Unlike other radical critics he does not see Alma Ata as a historic, revolutionary, progressive step.

46. Kenneth Newell, "Selective Primary Health Care: The Counter Revolution," *Social Science and Medicine* 26 (1988): 903–906.

47. Debabar Banerji, "Hidden Menace in the Universal Child Immunization Program," *International Journal of Health Services* 18 (1988): 293–299.

48. Wiener, "GOBI versus PHC?" 965.

49. Ibid., 966.

50. Ibid., 966.

51. Newell, "Selective Primary Health Care," 905.

52. Debabar Banerji, "Crash of the Immunization Program: Consequences of a Totalitarian Approach," *International Journal of Health Services* 20 (1990): 501–510.

53. Warren, "The Alma-Ata Declaration," 28. While Warren leaves his own role in the formation of the Task Force for Child Survival out of this article, in an interview he portrayed his role as much more active. Warren said that Salk came into his office and talked of going to see James Grant, head of UNICEF: "We were very upset by the slow pace of [WHO's] EPI [Expanded Programme on Immunization]. We had given up on them. We wanted a new organization. . . . We wanted Grant to focus the Children's Revolution on immunization" (interview with Warren, November 18, 1991). June Goodfield in her book *A Chance to Live: The Heroic Story of the Global Campaign to Immunize the World's Children* (New York: Macmillan, 1991) provides useful material on the establishment of the Task Force for Child Survival and Warren's role in it.

54. Interview with Warren, November 18, 1991.

55. Ibid.

56. Interview with Mahoney, April 29, 1991.

57. Memo by Mahoney, dated June 4, 1986, reporting on the meeting of May 29–30, 1986.

58. Interview with Mahoney, April 29, 1991.

59. Letter from Mahoney to Dr. S. Soewardjono, Minister of Health of Indonesia, September 5, 1986.

60. Memo by Mahoney, June 4, 1986, East Coast Trip Report #1, discussing the meeting with Task Force for Child Survival on June 2, 1986.

61. Interview with Warren, November 18, 1991.

62. Memo by Mahoney, June 4, 1986, Report #2, East Coast Trip, reporting on the June 2, 1986, meeting.

63. Ibid. In an interview with Mahoney (December 2, 1991), he said he felt

the creation of an ambitious but realistic protocol for the program and a carefully nurtured cooperation between the Task Force and PATH and the Indonesians in carrying it out. Fruitful collaboration required that the foreign team employ a suitable degree of tact and sensitivity when dealing with the elaborate etiquette of the Indonesian political and cultural systems. Unlike the initiators of many demonstration projects that had been established in the island republic, the Task Force did not try to impose its rules or values on the host culture. Rather, it accepted the established guidelines—though often adroitly maneuvering within them—in a manner consistent with Indonesian practice and sensibilities.

The Task Force quickly learned that there were innumerable unforeseen practical problems in attempting to immunize a large population of newborns within seven days of birth. However, with dedication, ingenuity, and the cooperation of key local individuals, the Task Force overcame nearly all of these problems. The Task Force discovered that flexibility was an indispensable requirement for working in Indonesia: it had to adjust its working procedures when they did not produce results, and it had to be willing to modify its ideals as well. One of the major commitments of the group was to foster community-wide, bottom-up participation to make the program self-sustaining. Its experience in the field, however, pointed in a different, less appealing direction. The Task Force discovered, much to its personnel's chagrin, that Indonesian society's commitment to hierarchy was so deeply ingrained that initiatives from the top were more likely to motivate villagers to cooperate than popular education or direct appeals to the people. Thus accepting and working within a cultural system that differed from its own conceptualizations, the Task Force nevertheless effectively supported its mission. The Task Force could, and did, continue to stress community outreach, but it substituted educating and persuading the local political leadership as its top priority. The Indonesian model also reinforced the Task Force's belief that a successful program required finding a national champion who would support the project against competitors and detractors. In Indonesia that role was played primarily by the Minister of Health, with the backing of the President of the Republic.

In the following pages we will see exactly how the Task Force's first model immunization project was able to change the world's attitude concerning the feasibility of fighting the hepatitis B pandemic.

*   *   *

The McDonnell Foundation proposal chose Indonesia as the site for the first model project for the Task Force. It was the inevitable choice because Richard Mahoney and PATH had been investigating the possibility of local production of hepatitis B vaccine there since the Minister of Health had raised the issue of liver cancer to them in 1984. Indeed, as we have seen, the driving force behind the formation of the Task Force was Mahoney and PATH's interest in Indonesia. To understand better what the Task Force accomplished in Indonesia it is necessary to begin by reviewing, in some detail, PATH's activities there before the Task Force was formed.

PATH Activities Preceding the Model Project

When PATH initially entered the hepatitis field in Indonesia in 1984 it found that most of the big pharmaceutical companies had already demonstrated an interest in either exporting vaccine or transferring the technology to produce it to Indonesia. The interested parties included the most important firms (Merck, Pasteur, SmithKline), as well as smaller groups (Korean Green Cross Corporation [KGCC], Biotech Corporation of Singapore,[1] the Dutch Red Cross). All of the companies were oriented toward the lucrative upper-middle-class/elite market, and all of the vaccines were too expensive to be usable in any type of mass immunization program.

PATH's mandate from the Minister of Health was to investigate the feasibility of establishing local production of a cheap vaccine, utilizable for just such large-scale vaccination projects. To assess the situation adequately, PATH had to make contact with those influential people, inside and outside of government, who were in a position to know both the opportunities and pitfalls facing such a venture.

In dealing with both private and public figures, PATH staff members were continuously challenged to employ all of the political savvy and cultural sensitivity they had painstakingly gained over the years they had operated in the country. Indonesia is a nation possessed of a long and powerful cultural-political tradition that forces people either to play by its rules or to find themselves excluded and ignored.

The system governing the country has been called a bureaucratic polity, which has meant that

the Indonesians have sought to gain security by agreeing that power should be hierarchically arranged so that each person can find his niche in a system of pyramided clusters of patrons and their individual clients. . . . [A]ll dormant power in society is concentrated in government hands. . . . At the heart of this bureaucratic polity is the idea of reciprocity between patron and clients.[2]

This bureaucratic arrangement, while characterized by the establishment of elaborate formal norms, has not given rise to orderly and efficient administrators oriented toward the achievement of some vital public purpose.[3] Rather, it has been shaped by a set of culturally unique rules and goals:

The Indonesian phenomenon of *bapakism*—consisting of a father figure, the *bapak*, and a circle of loyal followers called *anak buah* or children—is the cohesive glue which holds together the most intimate groupings in the bureaucracy.[4]

The links between important figures "may or may not follow the formal hierarchy of the bureaucracy,"[5] and as a result,

the Indonesian bureaucracy, in spite of its hierarchical appearance, is not one in which information and command flow smoothly and coherently between superior and subordinate offices. Rather, most offices, and even most officials at the same level, are often quite autonomous. . . . Therefore people . . . may not be well informed about a colleague's domain. . . . It is enough for all to pretend to knowledgeability with little expectation that they will ever be challenged.[6]

In this system, officials are primarily concerned with status, not the achievement of specific, practical goals:

Rarely does one try to find out what may be on the minds of others, but instead, one puts a positive gloss on what others are doing, almost as though that would bring about good relations with everyone. . . . Indonesians transform the bureaucratic game into one of protecting the status of the others. . . . Even high officials practice among themselves the Javanese art of . . . telling a person what he wants to hear. . . . The Javanese believes that it is better to tell another what will please him than to aggravate him with the truth.[7]

And as a result, there is

a bias in Indonesian politics against action and toward passivity. . . . [T]he ratio of speculation and rumor to hard evidence is higher in Jakarta than in most other political systems. Indonesians, who have a thirst for gossip, find genuine entertainment in talking about the activities of important figures.[8]

Outsiders who have wanted to know what is going on have had to sift carefully through the information they receive to assess its significance accurately.

The importance of the bureaucracy in Indonesia has meant that having the right client-patron relationship with government officials has been necessary for businessmen trying to establish viable private enterprises and indispensable for the achievement of real wealth.[9] Fortunately for entrepreneurs, President Suharto had "given scope to Western-trained technocrats who, as his clients, carefully treat him as their deserving patron"[10] and had looked favorably upon a growing number of client businessmen who received their start through government contracts. He had also given his blessing and protection to members of his family who wished to involve themselves in entrepreneurial pursuits.[11]

Vaccine Production and the Politics of the Quasi-Private Sector

PATH had to take these factors into consideration as it investigated the possibility for local manufacture of hepatitis B vaccine. It quickly discovered that there were two major entrepreneurs, Drs.[12] Wim Kalona, President of P. T. Darya Varia Laboratories, and Eddie Lembong, President and Director of P. T. Pharos, both with intimate ties to the Ministry of Health and significant experience in importing or producing vaccines. The two men proved vital sources of information on the economic and political landscape in Indonesia, though they mixed it with large amounts of rumor, unsubstantiated guesswork, and self-interested observations. For PATH the correct interpretation of the information it received was a formidable task.

Lembong of P. T. Pharos held very strong positions regarding what should and should not be done about hepatitis B production, and his contacts and experience made him a man whose opinions had to be respected. His ties to the Ministry of Health were close enough that he was the only private businessman included when the Minister of Health journeyed to Geneva for a 1986 conference. His firm was also the sole importer of SmithKline health products, and he imported a large variety of other medical products from a broad assortment of the best Western firms. Lembong told PATH that he knew of many exploratory contacts by foreign companies interested in vaccine production. Both SmithKline and the Wellcome Foundation had talked to him about transferring vaccine technology. He said that the Dutch Red Cross, South Korean firms, and Japanese companies, as well as a local foundation on the Indonesian island of Lombok, had all approached the Minister with proposals for local production of plasma-derived hepatitis B vaccine.

Several years earlier, Pasteur Vaccins had contacted BioFarma, the government pharmaceutical company, and offered to sell it its plasma vaccine. When BioFarma showed no interest, and the Merck company later contacted Lembong about its vaccine, he decided he could safely move ahead to import it himself. He sold it at $50 a dose ($150 for the series).

Despite the fact that he was engaged in selling Merck's plasma-derived vaccine, he believed that Indonesia should bypass it and use

Merck's new recombinant DNA vaccine. At the very least the country should avoid local production of plasma vaccine. Local plasma vaccine production, he contended, was impossible because adequate quality control could not be maintained. He warned PATH that he would use his considerable influence with the Minister of Health to discourage any plasma vaccine production.[13] As far as local recombinant DNA production was concerned, Lembong said that the Minister favored this process, and Lembong's company would be the logical producer of it. While it was true that BioFarma, as the state-owned pharmaceutical company, had the legal right to be sole producer, it would not do so because it was not an entrepreneurial-oriented organization, nor was hepatitis B high on its list of priorities. Besides, and more important, Lembong felt that his contacts in the Ministry were better than those of Dr. Nasution, the head of BioFarma.[14]

Lembong maintained that local vaccine production was only feasible if the government provided low-interest or interest-free loans. He recommended that PATH offer to provide a loan guarantee for the project if it were to be done through the private sector. He suggested a joint venture between the private sector and the government to finance production.[15] Lembong felt that it was vital that "no one will lose face,"[16] and thus a joint venture with BioFarma would be useful to serve that purpose.

Initially, to the PATH representative on the ground, Lembong's recombinant DNA ideas seemed reasonable. If the Minister supported it (and even Lembong's chief rival, Kalona, claimed that he did), then PATH should have a role in facilitating the transfer of technology since PATH always offered its clients a package that included technological and financial assistance.[17] The key problem for PATH was that its grant from the Bureau of Private Enterprise, U.S. Agency for International Development (USAID), specifically forbade any government involvement in ventures their money funded.[18] This was a supposedly pro-free market restriction that simply did not fit the facts of private entrepreneurship in Southeast Asia.

Independent of the funding problem, Mahoney by the late summer of 1985 had come to believe that recombinant DNA vaccine was totally impractical for Indonesia. By October 1985, PATH sent a letter to a close advisor to the Minister of Health saying that PATH opposed recombinant DNA vaccine production because of new quality control standards being discussed by the World Health Organization (WHO) which would make impossible even the first phase of production—the importation of bulk vaccine with local bottling and quality control.[19] This anti-recombinant DNA position, if nothing else, would have put PATH at odds with Lembong. The fact that his economic interests were deeply tied to the Merck company would also work to make him an enemy when PATH finally decided to concentrate its attention on the Cheil Sugar Company and its plasma vaccine.[20] However, in the interim his arguments were convincing enough to suggest a possible alternative strategy for PATH to follow:

[Lembong pushed a] theme: MSD [Merck] is sitting on a large supply of plasma vaccines and . . . they would lower the price if placed under some pressure (increasing competition). . . . The general idea is to capture the middle class market. . . . [H]e feels that getting at the lower public marke[t] . . . is economically not feasible in the foreseeable future. . . . [The creation of a] lower middle class marke[t] . . . would [ultimately] put pressure on the public sector and the vaccine manufacturers to work on eventual technological transfer leading to a[n] . . . affordable . . . DNA technology. . . . [It would] demonstrate the value of private enterprise in the vaccine field in Indonesia. . . . Lembong's motive is . . . to protect his share of the market . . . [but] this might be of real public benefit.[21]

Constructively working with Lembong, however, may have always been impossible because of a long-standing grievance that he had against PATH. PATH managed a number of different grants, some funded by philanthropic foundations and others by the U.S. federal government. Many of the programs had specific requirements that forced PATH to act in ways that limited its flexibility and undermined its explicit mission. Its USAID-funded Health Link program forbade any governmental involvement, which was counterproductive in most of Southeast Asia, and also required that PATH charge recipients of its grants fees for its services. Such a requirement seemed a reasonable way of stretching scarce funds so that more projects could be undertaken for the same amount of money. Unfortunately, fee-charging undermined PATH's image as a humanitarian, non-profit organization. Lembong had had dealings with another PATH program, the International Loan Fund, financed by the Ford Foundation, and he formed the opinion that PATH was simply a profit-oriented brokerage house for technical and financial services. That image would ultimately help sour his relationship with PATH over the hepatitis B vaccine.[22]

Lembong's misperception of PATH as a private money-making organization was unfortunately not unique, and such a view caused PATH a great deal of trouble at times, not only in Indonesia (and later in Thailand) but among certain U.S. governmental agencies as well. During the Reagan years there was a strong bias in favor of private enterprise (which PATH government contracts reflected) and a general suspicion of non-profit non-government-organizations, especially if they worked in the public sector. In the eyes of some Reagan appointees all such groups were Beltway bandits living off the federal government for the purpose of exploiting the taxpayer. PATH had to wage a continuous fight to counteract such unfavorable characterizations.[23]

PATH also had a problem of general philosophy with Lembong and other private entrepreneurs that was difficult to resolve. PATH's mandate in all its diverse Indonesian ventures was to strive to make health products more readily available, and at significantly lower prices. It often did this by aiding private companies. Its primary aim, however, was not to generate profits for an individual entrepreneur's sake, but to provide an inducement to get the product produced or imported at an affordable price. This approach may appear to create a conflict of interest: a representative of Lembong's company, when contacted about oral rehydration tablets, could not understand how PATH could have a relationship with one company and at the same time help its competitors. It looked to him as if PATH was perversely trying to increase competition and drive the price down. PATH's position that "healthy competition" helps improve quality and fair pricing was incomprehensible[24] from both an entrepreneurial and an Indonesian (client-patron) standpoint. In this case, PATH's ideals were in direct conflict with its commitment to be culturally sensitive to the people among whom it worked.

The other major businessman in pharmaceuticals in Indonesia was Kalona of P. T. Darya Varia. PATH found working with him much easier—because he had a strong interest in producing hepatitis diagnostic hardware and, later, producing hepatitis vaccine.[25] Even more important, unlike Lembong, Kalona was not yet committed to a foreign vaccine manufacturer. Kalona also had exceptionally good contacts in the government.

However, in initial discussion with Henry Wilde, Kalona took a decidedly negative position about local production of vaccine. He said discussions between KGCC and the Indonesian Red Cross had already taken place about starting a hepatitis B manufacturing plant, and that the government would exclude the private sector; thus, PATH was too late in entering the field. Despite Kalona's pessimistic view, which turned out to be based on a series of false rumors, it was clear to Wilde that Kalona was interested in producing the vaccine himself if it could be arranged.[26]

Kalona was quite adept at dealing with government officials, as he vividly demonstrated when the Minister of Health called together a group made up of individuals with an interest in hepatitis vaccines. The Minister's clear goal was to allow the airing of competing ideas and to reach some sort of consensus.[27] The Directors General of the Ministry of Health and other high-level staff were invited to this first meeting, along with only three private company representatives—among them Lembong and his rival Kalona. The head of BioFarma, Nasution, stated that the government pharmaceutical organization, while supportive of local efforts to produce hepatitis B vaccine, nevertheless considered measles and polio vaccine production its main priority. However, he added, if hepatitis B vaccine were locally produced, it could only be manufactured by BioFarma—a perfect example of catch-22, Indonesian style. Kalona, a master at bureaucratic politics, called Bio-Farma's bluff by saying that, if BioFarma officials wanted to produce hepatitis vaccine, he would personally "give" production to them.[28] He was quite aware that BioFarma had little desire to get involved in such a venture, and that they were frightened by its technical complexities, cost, and newness.[29]

As PATH's vaccine production investigations progressed and began to involve the possibility of transferring Cheil's plasma-derived vaccine technology to Indonesia, Kalona, unlike Lembong, was enthusiastic about participating. Kalona expressed a desire to represent Cheil in Indonesia, and PATH recommended him to Cheil[30] because of his experience, their good relations with him on other projects, and his close ties to the Minister of Health. By early 1986, PATH's game plan for Indonesia was premised on the assumption that Kalona and Cheil would cooperate. If they could not be successfully brought together, an entirely new strategy would need to be developed.[31] In the end an arrangement was made for Kalona to import the Cheil vaccine as part of a three-step plan that included (1) importation of the finished Korean vaccine, (2) importation of bulk vaccine that would be locally vialed (and subject to careful quality control), and (3) full-scale local production.[32]

PATH and Cheil Cooperate

In the months before the International Task Force on Hepatitis B Immunization was formed, PATH worked diligently for the Cheil vaccine. The Indonesian Minister of Health expressed support for the idea of transferring the Cheil/New York Blood Center plasma vaccine technology, but insisted that its Korean connection be hidden, and Kalona took the same position. The latter had agreed to use his considerable political clout to get Indonesian field trials for the vaccine started—even against the objection of the Director of Health Research and Development of the Ministry of Health, who favored a recombinant DNA vaccine. (It was speculated that the Director might have been swayed by extensive contact with SmithKline people, who were doing vaccine trials in Bandung, Indonesia, and promised a cheap vaccine by late 1986 or early 1987.)[33]

Cheil kept hearing rumors that other companies, especially its chief rival, KGCC, would beat it out in setting up production facilities. Cheil was especially afraid of an agreement between KGCC and BioFarma. Mahoney assured Cheil that this would not occur because the Cheil venture had the endorsement of the Minister and other key officials in the Ministry of Health—including the head of the Indonesian Food and Drug Administration and the Director of the Indonesian Communicable Diseases Control. In addition, Kalona had the political clout to keep all competitors out.[34]

Kalona used Cheil's fears as a tool to pressure the company to lower its price. Cheil, in the pre–Task Force period, wanted as high a price as it could get. Kalona felt if it were not careful it would price itself out of the middle-class market that he hoped to capture. Kalona believed the existing price was affordable only for the elite, and he hoped to lower it to $20 per adult dose and $10 per child dose, half the current price, to expand the number of those who could purchase it.[35]

Kalona's solution to the problem of KGCC-Cheil competition was to go to the relevant people and fix the price of the two vaccines (i.e, make arrangements to avoid price competition). PATH representatives were horrified at this solution. They actively discouraged him and warned him that if he was not careful his proposed price would match that charged by Pasteur, and his potential customers would buy the more prestigious French product. He was also cautioned that the new Taiwanese hepatitis B vaccine (the technology for which Pasteur was in the process of transferring) would be even cheaper and might flood the Indonesian market.[36] It was vital that Kalona sell at a lower price.

Ultimately, Kalona informed Cheil that he would find acceptable the same price at which KGCC was selling its vaccine, with the understanding that Cheil must match the price of any company that sold its product in Indonesia. He also told Cheil and PATH that he had been approached by "an exceptionally influential high ranking official"[37] who wanted to invest in the new hepatitis B manufacturing company. Kalona was already involved in other ventures with the same individual, and he was quick to inform the Minister of Health and the Director General of the Indonesian Food and Drug Administration about both the new company and the illustriousness of the shareholders in it. With such prestigious backing, Kalona told PATH, his position was greatly strengthened—though he emphasized that it was not appropriate to use the name of the individual to promote the company or its vaccine to the government (though simply passing information about it to key people seems to have been deemed legitimate).[38] Clearly the politics of vaccine production were intricate and required a sure and steady hand.[39]

The Benefits of a Local Intermediary

A key to PATH's success in Asia was its close relationships with politically astute individuals who could guide their efforts. The alliance with Kalona was one example of this. Even more important was PATH's relationship to one of Kalona's advisors, Dr. Anton Widjaya.[40]

Dr. Widjaya was a physician who worked for the Ministry of Health and advised P. T. Darya Varia, Kalona's company. He was both politically perceptive and a scientist in his own right. He was also one of the most well-informed men in Indonesia about the hepatitis B situation. Indeed, he was one of the first to alert the government to the magnitude of the problem.

Widjaya had been assigned to the island of Lombok in 1968 by the Ministry of Health and placed in charge of the provincial health laboratory. In 1972 he conducted a small survey of hepatitis B and reported to the Minister on what appeared to be significant findings. The Minister responded that nothing could be done about hepatitis B at that time. In 1975 Widjaya helped form a small group at the local hospital to further investigate hepatitis B on the island. The group carried out a study of governmental personnel and found rates of markers for hepatitis that equaled the highest ones found in Taiwan (where many of the landmark studies had been conducted). The results came as a rude shock, since there had been very little written or known about the disease in Indonesia. The group then proceeded to do a series of studies ranging from local children to military personnel. The results suggested that the problem on the island was severe and widespread.

When these studies were published they elicited significant interest from foreign scientists. A Japanese professor, Dr. Nishioka Kasuya, contacted Widjaya and offered to transfer technology for the preparation of hepatitis B diagnostic agents, which was a vital step if the situation in Indonesia was to be fully understood and successfully corrected. The Tokyo Metropolitan Institute of Medical Science paid for some staff members to go to Japan for the necessary training, and as a result the Lombok group was soon able to do laboratory-scale hepatitis B reagent production. The group then thought about expanding its work in two ways: (1) into commercial production of the diagnostic reagents and (2) later, into the production of hepatitis B vaccine. (This could be done because techniques for vaccine production build upon the skills learned for reagent manufacture.) Unfortunately, they encountered major obstacles that would prevent the achievement of either of those goals. First, the laboratory was mandated to provide service to the public, not to do research and production. Second, the government pharmaceutical organization (BioFarma) had a monopoly on the production of human vaccines.

To get around the first obstacle and perhaps ultimately the second, the group decided in the early 1980s to form a separate non-profit organization, the Healthy Liver Foundation. The Foundation initially received seed money from the local government in Lombok, and later obtained support from the Japanese, the Cancer Foundation, and the President of Indonesia.

Soon afterward Widjaya was transferred to Jakarta because he had already overstayed the normal rotation period for officials in a local placement. While in Jakarta he continued to work on improving the local (Lombok) production of reagents and looked into the possibility of vaccine production as well. He discovered that many officials in the capital and in Bandung (where BioFarma was located) were not only surprised at the work being done in Lombok but quite displeased by it. It was unusual in Indonesia for a laboratory/foundation to be far from the center of power. With the Japanese cooperating intensively in Lombok, government officials were feeling neglected and competitive.

In 1984 Widjaya had a chance meeting with Leona D'Agnes, the head of the small PATH office in Jakarta. Always on the look-out for new projects that involved technology transfer in the developing world, D'Agnes suggested the possibility of PATH's helping in the production of either hepatitis diagnostic reagents or vaccine production. It was at this point that hepatitis B became an area of potential interest for PATH—if not at the Seattle headquarters level, then at the local level. Widjaya was at that point hired as a consultant to PATH.

Widjaya and D'Agnes then proceeded to investigate the possibilities for PATH involvement in the hepatitis B area, though the issue was only one of a number of areas being considered, and it was placed only midway in the list of priorities.[41] PATH administered a sizable grant called Health Link, which focused on finding critical health problems and convincing private companies to work to solve them through the production or importation of appropriate technology. It seemed to D'Agnes that hepatitis B might fit the grant criteria.[42]

While it is not clear that this early local involvement with hepatitis B had any effect on Mahoney's subsequent intense interest in the issue (there is reason to believe that he did not even remember that he approved D'Agnes's request to bring Widjaya on as a consultant),[43] the vital relationship with Widjaya had already been firmly secured.

In Widjaya, PATH had a knowledgeable, diplomatic, and politically savvy individual who could serve as an intermediary between PATH and the government (and between PATH and Kalona's business empire). He could act as a conduit for information from PATH to the proper officials, and vice versa, while simultaneously working to smooth over conflicts and interpret communication in a way that harmonized the two groups. This is a vital function in every country, but especially in Indonesia, where avoidance of friction is highly valued. Widjaya could be sent to government officials to cut through politeness and ask them what real issues were at stake. On many occasions he delivered difficult messages to both sides[44]—messages that were hard to get across in a culture that strives to avoid saying or hearing negative information. A key function that Widjaya carried out was to alert PATH to potential trouble areas before they became disruptive, thus allowing time for PATH staff to discuss, explain, and defend their position. Early warning allowed PATH to prevent misunderstandings from getting into official documents, letters, or instructions that, once issued, might impede future cooperation or effectiveness.[45] Widjaya not only helped shepherd PATH/Task Force messages through the higher levels, he also helped the government "word their responses [in a way] that gives hope but doesn't make commitments,"[46] in keeping with the Indonesian communication style.

Widjaya's knowledge of Indonesia, public health, and hepatitis were invaluable enough that the hepatitis B model program in Indonesia might not have occurred without his aid. In planning the protocol that made the project feasible, and ultimately successful, his work was essential, as were his later reviews of the work-in-progress.[47] For example, at the start, when local Lombok health authorities made it known that they did not want the model project placed in their area—they did not want to fail at the field application of an impossible task—Widjaya went directly to the governor, whom he knew intimately, and obtained the aid necessary to elicit full and energetic cooperation from all lower official levels.[48]

Widjaya's aid constituted a major asset for PATH and, later, for the Task Force. But the fact that Widjaya wore "two hats" did create potential and actual conflict. When the question sometimes arose, "Who does Widjaya actually represent, the government or PATH and the Task Force?" the answer for Widjaya of necessity had to be the government. Some on the PATH staff were outraged when this happened and felt that this demonstrated his lack of loyalty. However, to higher-placed PATH/Task Force officers such as Mahoney, it was obvious that in a true conflict situation Widjaya had to act as the government's man. He could play no useful role for either the PATH/Task Force group or the government if he were seen primarily as an agent of an outside group. Widjaya's credibility depended on his primary loyalty to the Ministry of Health, thus demonstrating that mandatory loyalty did not conflict with his obligations as a PATH/Task Force advisor.

The Indonesian Minister of Health

Even more important to PATH and the Task Force's success in Indonesia as having skilled and influential men such as Widjaya and Kalona on their side was the unstinting support they received from the Minister of Health, Dr. S. Soewardjono. To achieve an ambitious program it was necessary to have a local champion, someone in a key agency that would fight the battles and make the work a cause.[49] Widjaya, for all his talents, was not powerful or important enough to fulfill that role.[50]

Mahoney realized quite early the importance of such an individual for the hepatitis B project because of his earlier work on a project involving contraceptives in Indonesia. In that case, President Suharto himself had established a national policy that the country would manufacture all the contraceptives needed for the Indonesian Family Planning Program. His personal intervention provided the bureaucracy with a clear mandate to cooperate. As a result, there was little difficulty in obtaining the necessary governmental approvals to set up the various factories and to import the required technical assistance.

Mahoney felt that if the Minister of Health could convince the President to take a similar role on this matter, the hepatitis B project's success would be assured. In this case, however, the Minister of Health himself was able to provide the power necessary to insure the success of the Lombok model project, though he lacked the influence to achieve the rapid movement toward local vaccine production that Mahoney also desired.[51]

Early on, when PATH staff people or Mahoney met with key government officials they encountered a great deal of resistance to taking action. Typical of this situation was Wilde's November 1985 meeting with Dr. M. Adhyatma, the powerful Director of Communicable Disease Control in the Ministry of Health. Wilde was presented with a barrage of reasons that hepatitis B could not be given either priority or fast-track action: the basic Expanded Programme for Immunization (EPI) vaccines were not being given to most children; there was not enough money to educate the public on health matters; there were not enough syringes for current vaccinations—they were either being used over and over again or illegally diverted to the private market; the cold chain required for vaccines was inadequate and the limited resources that existed were needed for polio and measles; high infant mortality due to diarrheal diseases, tetanus, or upper respiratory tract infections was more important; malaria was spreading. Hepatitis B could only be considered after all these other priorities were taken care of.[52]

In a similar vein Mahoney found a lack of enthusiasm when he met with the Directors General of the Ministry of Health and members of the Hepatitis B Advisory Committee in December 1985 and raised the issue of hepatitis B vaccine production. Dr. Loein, Head of the Research and Development Board, said it would take five years before Indonesia could produce a plasma-derived vaccine, and by that time the methodology would be outmoded. The transfer of plasma-derived vaccine technology was simply a fire sale of an old and soon-to-be obsolete technology. A hepatitis B program was too expensive and Indonesia could not afford a nationwide program. The other members of the meeting, with the sole exception of the head of the Indonesian Red Cross, wanted to move very slowly. In the absence of some countervailing force, there would have been nothing more PATH could have done to press its cause. There was never a lack of good and sufficient reasons to do nothing about hepatitis B—in Indonesia or anywhere else.

Although the Indonesian system of hierarchy did favor inaction, when the powers that be were really serious, the system could be effectively mobilized, and, fortunately, that proved to be the case with hepatitis B. The ultimate driving power behind the Minister of Health was President Suharto:

[In Indonesia] the president is the final arbiter in the Indonesian bureaucratic polity. . . . It is Suharto who decides who gets what share in return for supporting the president and his programs. . . . More than in most political systems, the personal beliefs of the chief executive leave their stamp on policy outcomes both large and small.[53]

In the case of hepatitis B, Suharto's concern was very strong and very personal—the death of a close associate, Foreign Minister Adam Malik, from liver cancer. This would have been enough by itself, given the system; his loss, however, was not unique, and that fact generated significant support among the elite, despite all the bureaucratic resistance. Even Dr. Adhyatma, Director of Communicable Disease Control, admitted to Wilde that notwithstanding the low priority he personally would give hepatitis B, the Ministry and Communicable Disease Control would be strongly pressured by important clinicians and politicians because of the deaths of several prominent political leaders from liver cancer.[54] A disease of middle-aged men that did not spare members of the ruling elite might be a silent epidemic to most people and appear to be less pressing than other ailments, but it nevertheless generated a potent constituency. Fortunately, their self-interested concern would work for the benefit of tens of thousands of future bread-winners who neither knew about the dangers that they faced nor had the power to initiate a protective program even if they did.

All of PATH's work investigating the possibility of local vaccine production, and all the contacts and alliances with local entrepreneurs and officials that it had forged over time, constituted the indispensable base that the Task Force would inherit when it entered the Indonesian arena.

PATH Acts as the Task Force's Indonesian Agent

The proposal the Task Force presented to the Indonesian government, unlike PATH's earlier work, subordinated the issue of local vaccine production to the idea of a large-scale model project that would demonstrate the feasibility of integrating hepatitis B vaccination into WHO's EPI—the foundation for any low-cost, mass hepatitis immunization program, and the key to obtaining a governmental commitment to a nationwide immunization program.

The first mention of establishing a model program in Indonesia came from D'Agnes, the head of PATH's Jakarta office, in 1985, a year before the Task Force was formed. She suggested the establishment of a two-phase program in either Thailand or Indonesia to begin large-scale testing of hepatitis B vaccine, perhaps supported by a USAID program.[55] James Maynard, who was then just learning about PATH, was told of her suggestion and responded enthusiastically; he immediately volunteered future Centers for Disease Control (CDC) aid in designing such a study at the point that it was funded by USAID or some other source. Maynard was himself a strong proponent of such an approach, and, as we have seen, he had been working to set up a similar project in Thailand. Though he was personally not familiar with the situation in Indonesia, D'Agnes's suggestion was consistent with his way of operating.[56] In an early conversation with Mahoney, he actually laid out a general plan for the introduction of local vaccine production that would be usable for any developing country. It included as a first step a pilot project lasting three to five years in which a target group would be vaccinated, doctors trained, Ministry of Health officials educated, and the most efficient way to operate the vaccine delivery system developed. He believed one did not just rush into vaccine production.

Once the Task Force was formed and its proposal to do a project in Indonesia was accepted, Maynard, as Chief of the Hepatitis Branch of the CDC, was in a perfect position to lend active support to the Task

Force and the Indonesian government. He and a member of his staff, Dr. Fred Shaw, flew to Indonesia to help write the protocol for the model program, and they produced what turned out to be the framework for the proposal.[57]

Vaccine Price for the Model Project

The ability to carry out a demonstration project in Indonesia successfully would depend on many factors, but the most important one was obtaining sufficient supplies of vaccine at an affordable price. The Task Force did have Cheil's general commitment to the $1-per-dose price, though for purposes of the pilot project the pledge had little practical significance since Cheil required a minimum of five million doses to trigger the price.[58]

It is interesting that the problem of getting Cheil to pledge itself to $1 per dose—a price favored by the Task Force and PATH-Seattle—initially caused a great deal of consternation in the local PATH office in Jakarta. PATH had spent a great deal of time and effort setting up a relationship between Cheil and the pharmaceutical entrepreneur Kalona. An agreement was reached between him and Cheil that he would first import and later locally produce hepatitis B vaccine. The price would be lower than existing prices, but still substantial enough to be affordable only for the growing middle class. The Task Force's talk of $1 per dose threatened to undercut the market for such a venture. Kalona made it clear to D'Agnes that he did not look favorably on such Task Force involvement in Indonesia. Even the Minister of Health, whose goodwill was crucial to the Task Force, expressed some anxiety that such a low price from Cheil might undercut the possibility of successful local production, a goal he strongly supported because of its role in advancing the technological development of the country. D'Agnes felt that talking up the idea of a $1-dose ran the risk of raising expectations without being able to deliver on them (Cheil kept procrastinating on making its offer firm and insisted that the price might not prove to be economically feasible). Even if Cheil did firmly commit itself to the low price, it would surely kill Kalona's local production venture, since he would not be able to match it. Such a situation would lead to frustration and hostility for both the public and the key decision makers.[59]

Despite the complications that the new model program might cause for existing arrangements, the Task Force absolutely needed the $1-per-dose benchmark to make its work possible. To achieve the price, it could have simply negotiated with Cheil to supply the vaccine to the project, but the Task Force wanted more than a cheap price for the first project. It wanted to establish a precedent that would support mass immunization in the future for all public projects. So, rather than negotiating with Cheil, the Task Force in 1987 recommended to the Indonesian government that a sealed international bid and tender be set up that would allow all hepatitis B vaccine manufacturers registered in Indonesia to compete for the contract to supply the vaccine. For most members of the Task Force this was seen as just a formality. Cheil would of course underbid everyone else, though it would establish a reasonable procedure for other countries.

The Task Force had originally raised the issue of a bid and tender with the major pharmaceutical companies when it invited them to attend the Task Force's first formal organizational meeting in Nairobi, Kenya, in March 1987.[60] At that time it discussed the preliminary criteria it would require. It was doubtful that all companies would actually be willing to compete, since a representative of SmithKline stated that his company would not bid "because it would be very embarrassing to lose to a Korean manufacturer."[61] The Task Force knew that many Western companies felt it was a matter of pride and prestige that they charged more than the Asian companies.[62]

The result, however, was quite unexpected. The bid and tender attracted many companies—Western and Asian—including SmithKline. Everyone offered the vaccine at prices considerably below what they were selling for up until that point. The formal bidding procedure forced many companies to begin to think about the possibility of significant price reductions, though most of the lower prices were still too high for any mass immunization campaign.

Surprisingly, the lowest bid did not come from Cheil, but from its chief competitor, KGCC, which offered to supply the vaccine at $0.95 a dose. Thus the $1-a-dose requirement was not only met but broken. In addition, it was not presented by the bidder as a humanitarian or philanthropic gesture, but rather as a straightforward business proposition. In reality, the KGCC bid broke the price of hepatitis B vaccine in a way that the original Cheil offer had not. When Chairman B. C. Lee of the Samsung group (which owned Cheil) made his $1-a-dose offer, it was based on the assertion that the vaccine would be more expensive to produce and would require his personal subsidy to achieve the low price.[63] KGCC's offer was a straight-out profit-making $0.95, no subsidy included.

Not only was KGCC willing to go below $1 a dose, it was also willing to meet a key bid requirement: "The bidder shall commit to provide vaccine at the same price to other public sector agencies for similar quantities . . . [and] also commit to filling future needs of the Task Force for the Indonesian program at the same price."[64] This was vital for the Task Force: maintaining the price for large-scale public purchases and preventing dumping of the vaccine by companies for purposes of gaining prestige (to be followed up by much higher prices).[65] The Task Force's goal was to be seen as providing "the Good Housekeeping Seal" for vaccines, and it did not want the seal bought by a company willing to bid at a price lower than what it would give to other purchasers.[66]

Such a position was very important for precedent setting. It was also significant, since Cheil responded to the underbidding by attempting just such an unacceptable maneuver. Shin Seung-il of Cheil communicated that Chairman Lee of Samsung wanted to reiterate his commitment to the hepatitis B program, and he "has proposed to provide personal cash subsidies, the amount of which shall be equivalent to one half of the delivered cost of the Cheil vaccine."[67] He would go so far as to provide subsidies for the first million doses—with the possibility of extension.

The Task Force responded that it "would be delighted to get the contribution, but not contingent"[68] upon giving Cheil the initial Indonesia vaccine order. The award was based upon sealed bids and could not be changed afterward. The whole situation was exceptionally beneficial for the Task Force. As Alfred Prince saw it,

KGCC underbid Cheil. We were sensitive [to the possibilities inherent in this]. We did not want to be seen as Cheil's representative. . . . Mr. Lee of Samsung's half charity [letter] was rejected because it was not offered to all and looked like he was "buying" us. We did not want a sweetheart price and [then have them] using us to tell the world how great they were. We wanted to set the price. We were in the driver's seat—[something] unusual for people like us. We wanted to use our clout.[69]

The whole question of vaccine subsidies and donations was a sensitive issue for the Task Force. Insofar as its goal was to force the international price of hepatitis B vaccine down, it was necessary to foster competitive pricing. There was the temptation, however, to get free vaccine to stretch the Task Force's financial resources and accomplish its other goals. Ian Gust, the conscience of the group and one of its most outspoken members, was vehemently opposed to accepting vaccine donations at all. He wanted the price permanently lowered. On more than one occasion internal debates became rather heated over this issue. For the first couple of years of its existence the Task Force refused donations. Later, it accepted them but only on condition that the manufacturer stated it would sell vaccines at less than $1 a dose on subsequent occasions.[70] (One of the chief strengths of the Task Force was that it could tolerate adamant positions and heated debate without grudges or fissures developing in their wake.)

For many on the Task Force, surprise at KGCC's bid was mixed with pleasure and relief because the true disinterestedness and impartiality of the group could finally be clearly demonstrated. This is not to say that there was not initial dissent. The Cheil vaccine was Prince's creation, and he had a strong belief that it was the perfect vaccine for the developing world. He did not like aspects of the KGCC production process, which he considered inferior, and was initially reluctant to accept the KGCC bid. In addition, Shin Seung-il claimed that KGCC had altered its process recently and this had adversely affected its product. However, these objections were dealt with in turn, and the offer was accepted.[71]

As an interesting aside on the complexity of pharmaceutical competition, the KGCC begged the Task Force not to announce publicly what their winning bid was. They said they were afraid of the effect of such information on both their normal market and their business relations with other commercial companies.[72] They did not want to anger their competitors. Of course the Task Force could not agree to such a request since the low price was a major weapon in its bid to have other companies follow suit. Secrecy about the winning bid was the last thing it wanted. In the eyes of Task Force members such as Gust, the result of the formal bid and tender was an accomplishment of historic proportions. The unsubsidized low price demonstrated that if a mass market was created an affordable price could be achieved. Even if the Task Force had disbanded on the day the bids came in, it would have accomplished its primary goal of making large-scale hepatitis B immunization economically feasible. The sealed bid and tender, followed by the public announcement of the winning offer, broke the price of the vaccine and removed the chief obstacle to an effective war against hepatitis B.[73]

The Indonesian Model Project

The Task Force had decided to achieve something much more ambitious than simply lowering the price of the vaccine. It was determined to establish a model project that definitively proved hepatitis B could be successfully integrated into the existing EPI of WHO.

The site chosen for the model program was the island of Lombok, which was in one of the poorer provinces of Indonesia. On its own the Task Force would not have voluntarily chosen Lombok as its demonstration area because of the area's noticeably poor EPI coverage.[74]

Adding a new vaccine in such an area would be a more difficult task than it would be elsewhere, thereby potentially lowering the chance of success. However, the Minister of Health personally recommended Lombok because of the Healthy Liver Foundation and laboratory that Widjaya and others had established there and the long-standing concern of the local doctors and the island's Governor about hepatitis B. Without their interest and work the national government would not have been aware of the problem in the first place, nor would have the Minister himself. As it turned out, Lombok was a fortunate choice, because by proving success was possible there, the Task Force demonstrated it was possible anywhere in Indonesia.[75]

To facilitate the project the government appointed two teams: a National Team, headed by the Minister of Health, and a Provincial Team, headed by the Principal Investigator. The Task Force appointed Ian Gust of Australia to act as Monitor for the program and to make periodic inspections of the work. The Task Force was also represented by a local full-time representative on Lombok, Brad Otto, who had previously worked at the U.S. CDC. Significantly, the Jakarta PATH office and its staff functioned as the Task Force's general agent.

The Protocol

The protocol for the demonstration project was hammered out over a period of months during 1987. It was vital that the protocol be as clear, concise, and accurately detailed (with well-thought-out indicators to measure success and failure) as possible, because a positive outcome for such projects largely depends on the original plan's quality and the degree to which it can be implemented. The protocol was developed primarily under the guidance of Maynard, drawing upon assistance from CDC personnel. PATH acted primarily as an intermediary between Maynard's people and the Indonesians.[76] Detailed knowledge of the island of Lombok came from PATH and their team on the site. They then sat down with the Ministry of Health people in the field. Subsequently, the U.S. CDC personnel worked on the draft with D'Agnes and members of the National Indonesian Team. It took more than four months to produce a satisfactory document, after which the protocol was sent through a number of governmental levels (Ministry of Health, Ministry of International Affairs, and so on up the line) and further embellished. Passage through the different levels of bureaucracy took a great deal of time (a full year) before everyone agreed on the protocol.[77]

The final product of their work was "A Model Immunization Program for Hepatitis B in Lombok, Indonesia: Protocol," presented to the Ministry of Health by the Task Force and PATH in May 1987. It proved to be an exceptionally sound foundation from which to begin their work.

The stated goal of the protocol was to "attempt to identify obstacles in the delivery of hepatitis B vaccine to newborns"[78] as a model not only for Indonesia but all developing countries. It firmly stated that the investigation was aimed at integrating hepatitis B immunization into the existing EPI. The protocol stated that a major factor that made Lombok a desirable site for the model was the existence of a core of deeply committed physicians on the island who had a long-term interest in hepatitis:

Several of these physicians, led by Drs. Soewignjo, Widjaya [et al.] . . . had recognized the problem of hepatitis B-induced chronic liver disease in Lombok . . . [and] with [the] assistance of the Provincial Governor, . . . had established a Foundation for the study and treatment of hepatitis B and had constructed a modern . . . laboratory specifically dedicated to hepatitis B diagnosis and therapy.[79]

The document presented the vital statistics of the chosen site, including the social, economic, and political realities that of necessity shape all health interventions: (1) Lombok was an island with a population of 2.3 million, most of whom were ethnic Sasaks who practiced Islam. About 40 percent of the population could not read or write Bahasa Indonesian, the national language. Daily conversation was in Sasak, and per capita income was $82 a year. Over 90 percent of births occurred at home, with the vast majority involving traditional birth attendants, most of whom were illiterate.[80] (2) The political structure of the province was headed by the Provincial Governor. The province was divided into three districts, each headed by a leader called a *Bupati*. Districts were in turn divided into subdistricts, headed by a *Camat*. Under the *Camat* was the village head, a respected man in the village who may or may not be a government employee. At the sub-village level was a hamlet chief, who was the central figure in the life of the hamlet.[81] (3) The Indonesian Village Women's Movement (PKK) played a vital role in delivery of EPI vaccines. The Ministry of Health encouraged the PKK to motivate and educate mothers who had children in need of vaccination. The PKK organization's structure paralleled the political structure: The PKK leader at every level was the wife of the political leader. (In Lombok, however, the PKK members were not fully organized and trained to be motivators.)[82] (4) By Indonesian law all births had to be officially registered within forty-eight hours of the birth, though in practice only 40–50 percent were officially registered.[83] (5) The health system was built around forty-eight stationary centers that delivered a wide range of services. They in turn provided periodic outreach services to the villages and hamlets, of which there were 850. These clinics were held approximately every one to three months at the house of a prominent individual. They usually involved a vaccinator, but not a physician. The outreach service was primarily passive; people were required to seek it out. In much of Lombok, vaccinations were offered only after a baby reached three months of age. Delivery of EPI vaccines depended heavily on the vaccinators, most of whom were not formally educated in a health discipline but received a three-month apprenticeship training.[84] (6) Approximately 10 percent of the general population were hepatitis B carriers. Between 20 and 30 percent of hepatitis virus infection passed from mother to child; the rest of the cases occurred via horizontal transmission between children.[85]

Against this background, the protocol laid out the project's objectives. First,

all operations relating to the delivery of hepatitis vaccine [will] be integrated with the delivery of . . . EPI vaccines. As far as is possible, no project activity will be directed solely toward the delivery of hepatitis B vaccine . . . [and] . . . the methods used in the project [should] be replicable to other regions of Indonesia and other developing countries. It is hoped that this project will stimulate the adoption of childhood hepatitis B immunization for all of Indonesia.[86]

In meeting this objective, the project would attempt to achieve a 65 percent success rate in delivering three doses of hepatitis B vaccine to children under fifteen months, and in the same time frame achieve a 60 percent success rate in delivering all EPI vaccines to children under fifteen months in eighteen evaluation ("core") villages, which would be selected.

Another objective of the project would be to identify the major practical obstacles to administering hepatitis B vaccine within seven days of birth to infants born in their homes. While doing this, personnel would also study the effectiveness of off-schedule versus on-schedule vaccination as well as factors affecting parents' acceptance of newborn vaccination at home.[87] The project would attempt to achieve a 75 percent success rate in reporting births to the village chief within forty-eight hours and study methods of sterilizing vaccination needles.

The program, according to the protocol, would be managed by a dual team composed of representatives of the International Task Force on Hepatitis B Immunization and PATH on one side and members of the Indonesian National Team on the other side. The National Team would be represented in Lombok by a Provincial Team, whose leader would be the Principal Investigator.[88]

The protocol assumed that members of the PKK would perform

vital roles in notifying the village heads of birth and carrying out a call-back system to make sure that infants received the second and third vaccinations.[89] In addition, a special notification system would be set up outside of the official registration channels.[90]

To evaluate the effectiveness of the program, a serologic and immunization survey would be performed in the eighteen selected core villages before the start of the project (to create a baseline) and at the end of the second and fourth years (to test if carriership and infection rates had actually declined).[91]

The protocol treated education and training activities as vital and indispensable parts of the project. Education would be aimed at the political organization, the health administration, the PKK, and pregnant mothers.[92]

The possibility of successfully carrying out the protocol was vastly increased when the Minister of Health, in an unusual gesture, issued a Special Decree for the project. The rarity of such decrees gave the project extremely high status, something "very important and essential in Indonesian politics."[93] In addition, the project leaders were given authority to implement changes, when needed, in other ongoing Ministry of Health programs that existed in Lombok (e.g., birth registration, outreach vaccinator schedules). Giving such power even to government groups was almost unheard of in Indonesia. Project leaders also had the right to change key elements of their program as they went along. This provided them with an uncommon amount of flexibility, especially in a country that had elaborate bureaucratic rules that discouraged independent action.[94] The government was clearly giving them permission to model "an approach"[95] that would be followed elsewhere in the country. This was a real coup for the Task Force—and an absolutely necessary one, since constant checking, rechecking, and adjustments to field conditions were indispensable for the project's success. Such flexibility was also the hallmark of PATH's methodology, upon which the Task Force relied.

The Need for Cultural Sensitivity

Successful implementation of the project required a great deal of political and cultural awareness on the part of PATH and Task Force personnel. According to D'Agnes the project involved co-governance by the Task Force/PATH and the National/Provincial Teams.[96] The protocol officially concentrated all responsibility for the program, however, only in the hands of the National Team. The Task Force's full-time local representative (the Counterpart Project Officer, Brad Otto) was given no direct operational authority; such authority resided only with the Principal Investigator. While Otto was allowed to consult directly with the PATH office in Jakarta as needed, a copy of any formal written communications had to be sent to the National and Provincial Teams.[97]

The nature of Indonesian politics and culture required the official line of authority to be lopsided in this way. The reality needed to be, and was, quite different. Successful co-governance meant very careful operation. As D'Agnes put it:

You had to give all credit to the government [team]. They have to look like they do everything, though it is really shared. On the organizational chart we never directly communicate with the Principal Investigator. We officially communicate [only] through the National Team to the Provincial Team. In Indonesia this [formal] chart flow is vital. [In reality] on a personal level we go to individual members of the National Team. I go and say "there is a problem with finance etc." but in all written documents it is done differently: it shows who should communicate with whom—[the required] protocol.[98]

PATH people like D'Agnes knew the members of the National Team personally and knew the culturally correct ways of dealing with them from the decade or more of experience PATH had in Indonesia.[99] When Otto, the Task Force's full-time representative in Lombok, arrived he quickly discovered that sensitive political issues, especially negative aspects of the work, could not be written down because his Provincial Team colleagues would be offended. When he relayed problems to PATH-Jakarta, he had to keep his communications oral and informal.

When PKK, an important group favored by the government, was found inadequate for its vital role, it could not be openly criticized and replaced, but rather was unofficially "supplemented" by alternative sources.[100] D'Agnes noted that there was a set of unwritten rules that had to be carefully followed if good relations were to be maintained:

The Ministry of Health is our host—we have to be diplomatic. We don't hide things. They respect that . . . we are careful not to confront them. We can [in fact] confront them but [only] in a non-confrontational way. . . . We [always] link bad new with good[;] . . . [give] gentle reminders of what needs to be done (not attacks for not doing it); . . . [and] tell . . . them how things can go smoothly. All this softens the blow. [We] never begin a letter [to an official] with a negative. Some Americans are against diplomacy [and say] "do it our way or we will leave." You can be more straightforward in direct talks, [in] closed session, than on paper. One to one you can [actually] confront a person . . . but [you] can't do [it] if a witness is present or in writing.[101]

Sensitivity to such nuances was vital for the Task Force's project to have any chance of succeeding. D'Agnes was even careful regarding what kinds of background information she put in writing to PATH headquarters in Seattle for fear that visitors from Seattle would drop the information in conversation with government officials without realizing it might be damaging.[102]

The Vital Role of Educational Materials

In the months before the protocol was submitted, and in the years after it was approved, PATH and Task Force personnel were busy developing instruments to carry out the project, and checking and rechecking for possible weaknesses in them. PATH, in keeping with its long-standing exactitude in designing culturally appropriate educational materials for pre- and semiliterate people, was especially concerned with the quality of its manuals and instructional materials.

To obtain information for inclusion in the teaching manuals, PATH made use of Focus Group Discussions (FGDs), which brought together representatives of selected populations to find out their concerns, perceptions, and misconceptions regarding key issues. The FGDs demanded great delicacy on the part of the discussion leaders in order to be effective; if it was not forthcoming the work was rejected and done over again. For PATH, conducting the research properly was fundamental:

In terms of identifying a group to conduct the FGDs, it is very important that the facilitators be sensitive to the need to listen much more than they speak, that they understand the kinds of information we are seeking, and that they probe for it in a nondirective way.[103]

According to D'Agnes the creation of successful educational materials took painstaking effort: "Our experience is that print materials need to be pretested [with the target population] and modified at least twice, to come up with an acceptable product."[104] Anything less would not do.

One of PATH's key tasks was to make sure that the assumptions in the protocol proved correct, and that its directives were practical in the field. Constant checks on progress and practicality were built into the program; nothing was to be taken for granted. The same care was taken with all instruments designed to further the project.

One of the first places this technique proved itself was in the design of the project's logo. During a series of FGDs with village women designed to find out what the villagers knew about disease and immunization, and to discover images that would appeal to the population, the idea for a project symbol was developed. In preparing the logo, the designers drew a cartoon of a young boy crouched behind a shield and clutching a bamboo rod. The shield was emblazoned with a syringe to symbolize that injections acted like a shield to protect the child. The logo was very appealing to the designers, but when it was pretested in nonproject areas "the consensus of women . . . was that the crouching boy was hiding behind the shield because he was embarrassed by his nakedness."[105] The designers immediately discarded the cartoon and searched for a more culturally appropriate symbol—ultimately using a popular figure from local stories.

The Protocol Is Modified by Reality

The protocol, like the instruments designed to further it, required significant revision as the project unfolded. Assumptions built into it were continually tested for accuracy and when found wanting were revised. In a PATH internal document some vital flaws in the initial proposal were indeed discovered:

[The] village layout is often much less convenient than is suggested by the schematic village map included in the project protocol. One village in which we worked . . . is long and skinny, stretching about 30 kilometers from end to end. It is cut by deep, unbridged ravines all along its length. There is no way that a vaccinator could follow the protocol . . . [and that village] is not untypical.[106]

A larger problem was uncovered when they investigated the vital question of birth notification:

Regarding use of the PKK [the Women's Movement, which the government required them to employ] for birth notification: when we pretested pictures of PKK workers in some villages, illiterate villagers often said "who?" We learned that even though there may be a chart showing existence of a PKK infrastructure [in the local leader's] . . . office, villagers may haven no idea of what the PKK is or who their PKK member is (if indeed she exists at all).[107]

Things were no better in regard to the local vaccinators:

In almost every health center we visited, we found vaccinators [for the EPI vaccines]. They are supposed to spend only one or two days there . . . yet we found them with free time to work with us on "field days." We did not see any of them vaccinating. This observation clearly supports villager claims that they do not see vaccinators as often as we might hope.[108]

Most dangerous of all was the general attitude they found among their local health worker allies:

[Concerning the] reporting of negative results . . . there is a strong cultural reluctance to report negative results. This program will be a success, even if it is not. It will be difficult to obtain, document, and release objective evaluation data. We (PATH) are only supposed to see what works and local staff go to great length to try to ensure that this happens.[109]

The challenge to PATH and the Task Force was to find solutions to these pressing problems and to adjust the protocol so that it could work even under such adverse conditions.

Exactly how careful one had to be not to offend Indonesian sensibilities was illustrated when the results of the first FGDs conducted with vaccinators were evaluated. The National Team staff members were mortified because they felt that what the vaccinators said about disease causation demonstrated extreme ignorance. They feared the results, if disseminated, would reflect disastrously on their field staff. The National Team did not understand that the official purpose of those discussion groups was to elicit vaccinator perceptions of popular beliefs, not their own personal perceptions. (PATH staff people who tried to explain this fact to the National Team were themselves privately afraid that "the [exceptionally detailed] level of knowledge of vaccinators regarding folk remedies and spiritual causation [of disease] suggests that they themselves may [indeed] subscribe to many of these beliefs and may practice traditional healing."[110] This fear was diplomatically excluded from the written analysis of the FGD results.)

The recommendation to PATH personnel that came out of the National Team/PATH interactions was to "keep these cultural constraints in mind when developing evaluation protocol . . . be very tactful in reporting anything that is not working as well as it should . . . [and] in future discussion with national and provincial staff, [strongly] emphasize that this is a pilot project which seeks to uncover system problems in order to address them in the future"[111] and thus defuse any possible embarrassment.

To make sure that the educational material they were producing would serve its purpose, and that their evaluation of field problems was as accurate as possible, PATH brought in an outside expert who had intimate knowledge of administrative structures, organizations, and capabilities of personnel at various administrative levels in Lombok, and who was comfortable receiving input and information from field staff. His analysis of the Vaccinator Manual pointed out:

[A key part of it] doesn't get at the problem of inaccurate reporting of positive results to please superiors. There is little emphasis on the problems encountered and correctly reporting these so that the program might change to accommodate the needs of the people.[112]

More importantly he emphasized the problem of relying upon the PKK to motivate mothers and register births. He explained that the PKK was required by the government to carry out many different programs in addition to the hepatitis project, and that every day they spent doing that work was a day without working for a living. He reported that local doctors at the health centers told him that PKK members were motivated only in those programs that provided incentives, and that even the best programs and strategies were useless if not adequately motivated. The expert felt that inducements were necessary. He suggested that incentives could be structured so they did not lead to excessive costs, and argued that strategies for motivating people had to receive as much attention as that given to training, serologic surveys, and other traditional "vital" tasks.

The PKK Creates a Crisis in the Field

Offering incentives was in keeping with both PATH and the Task Force's way of looking at things. Unfortunately, it ultimately became clear that the PKK, even with incentives, was not capable of carrying out the vital role the project and the government required of it. This created a major crisis for the Task Force. The government demanded that the PKK be the chief instrument of the project, and this mandate could not be openly denied or officially changed. But the project would not succeed if it relied upon the PKK:

We couldn't drop the Women's Movement [PKK] no matter how poorly they did. That is politics. . . . It is more than saving face. Women are terribly overburdened in mobilizing community participation for many issues, not just health. No blame on them. We at headquarters have to put a reality check on ideals of what can be done. We have to work around the reality.[113]

The reality that had to be worked around was extremely difficult. On paper, the PKK was a highly organized, hierarchic, and prestigious force made up of the wives of political leaders at every governmental level. But the actual village situation was quite different:

They [PKK members] are volunteers. [They receive] no pay. They end up being teenage girls ([and] some boys) without children, jobs etc. In Lombok they are often illiterate. They are young and not respected members of the community. They leave when they get married—they marry-out and [thus] leave the village.[114]

The way to get around this problem was to supplement the system unofficially. PATH tried to get hamlet chiefs, parents, and traditional birth attendants to fill in the gaps. The traditional birth attendants were seen as especially attractive since they were present at most births. Unfortunately, the government considered them "untouchables" (because they were elderly, illiterate women) and was reluctant to involve them or train them. Over time the Ministry of Health became more receptive to the idea of using the attendants, but by then it was too late to incorporate them into the official structure.[115] Over the course of the project's duration, PATH was never able to find an adequate substitute for the PKK. But the project teams, by using official and unofficial sources for birth notification, were able to achieve a remarkably high coverage rate—70 percent in the first week after birth, which was only slightly below the 80 percent level they had hoped for under ideal conditions.[116]

One of the tools utilized by the Task Force and PATH was the provision of monetary and in-kind incentives. This strategy had been recommended not only by PATH's outside expert's report, but also by the Ministry of Health itself. The most important incentive was travel money or its equivalent (gasoline, or a vehicle). The government did not usually provide such resources, which was why the government health service did not reach below the village administrative level, to the hamlets where most rural people lived. Without travel incentives, the health system let (or forced) people to come to it—often from great distances. Community leaders such as the hamlet chiefs technically were required to go to the village to report births. The Task Force and PATH provided money to fund their travel. If they walked, they could keep the money as compensation for the extra work. Other non-governmental organizations criticized PATH for giving the monetary incentives, but PATH felt it needed to be done. Adopting the monetary award incentives would be cost effective for the government, if not immediately, then in the future when multiple services (e.g., hepatitis B vaccination, polio vaccination, vitamin A supplements) would be delivered together.[117]

Overcoming Cultural Obstacles to Long-Term Success

The Task Force's goal in setting up the model project was to demonstrate that a mass hepatitis B immunization program was possible and to inspire Indonesia and other countries to establish national programs. In keeping with this goal, it was important that the project in Lombok be seen not as a temporary activity (i.e., a one-shot "vertical" program), but as a sustainable enterprise, integrated with other ongoing health programs. As Brad Otto noted, it was very difficult to convince key people in the villages to adopt this perspective because

projects here are traditionally seen as short term, despite donor wishes. They aren't seen as sustained issues. They have time limits. Then they go back to the way they have done before. We try to convince people that this is to be integrated into [WHO's] EPI. This has been extremely difficult to get fixed in the local team (in the local health center). They are used to seeing one or two year WHO or UNICEF studies.[118]

D'Agnes was very aware that the "short term project is easy [but] institutionalization is the hard part."[119] Over the years she had seen "so many quickies with 'social marketing' that they then claim[ed] were successful but long-term were not,"[120] she was determined not to fall into the same trap. She was not opposed to utilizing such techniques—they were vital—but she believed they had to be embodied in a long-term commitment.[121]

If the "temporary project" mindset was fostered by the activities of non-Indonesian organizations, it was even more influenced by the nature of Indonesian society and government. As Otto observed:

Indonesian society is fairly patriarchal—people especially in the Civil Service do what they are told. They are not given the opportunity to assess what they are told. This makes the idea of sustainability hard. We [PATH and the Task Force] try to work from the bottom up—from local people to the province, etc. We try to get their vision of the constraints and problems. [But] that is like pulling teeth. We can't get [their] view. Quarterly reports tell of the same weaknesses year after year—no solutions offered. No initiatives, no imagination on how to overcome these constraints.[122]

The reason they do not help is that "they don't see it as their role to change or improve things";[123] rather, they see this as the responsibility of those higher up in the hierarchy. This attitude is not restricted to bureaucrats. Among the general population too "[t]here is a strong reliance on village leaders and vaccinators to tell them when and where to report for the next immunization session rather than on their own feelings of personal responsibility."[124]

To succeed the Task Force and PATH had to adapt to the real conditions it found in the field:

[This lack of local initiative] is cultural. We can't do anything [about it]. We try to overcome this by having good relations with the higher levels. We had very good relations with the Governor. . . . He issued decrees that made it possible for lower levels just to follow orders. . . . Working with District Chiefs and their wives [and their equivalents at lower levels] we spend a lot of time cultivating . . . relations—to overcome the lack of initiative from below by giving decrees that subordinates can "just follow." [It takes] a lot of effort.[125]

The Task Force found that the official decrees, whether issued by the Minister of Health, the Governor, or the local leaders, were not meaningless, since they quickly brought dramatic results. Local people would cite the decree and then cooperate. The top-down approach was not what the Task Force or PATH preferred—indeed, critics of immunization programs would probably find this acceptance of the existing social/cultural situation appalling—but without such an accommodation the demonstration project would have failed, and the possibility of a nationwide immunization program would have been lost.

Because official cooperation was required to initiate action, it became obvious that producing health education to the leadership cadre had to take precedence over parental education:

At PATH we are very education-oriented: let people make [their own] choices. In Indonesia [the] very elaborate hierarchic structure meant we did not have to explain why people should be immunized—it was very clear that officials had to be educated and people would follow. [Nevertheless] we tried to find a middle way. . . . We worked through the PKK. . . . We are looking to work with other institutions like religion. We have gone to radio. . . . [However, printed] pamphlets are for leaders and PKK, not parents, [though] there were parent[-oriented] booklets in the first year.[126]

Although the leadership-oriented approach was very hard for PATH and its staff to accept—since it ran counter to their democratic ideals, their sense of progressive community service, and their vision of themselves as innovative educational providers—the importance of educating the leadership cadre became one of the key lessons learned from the Lombok project. This strategy was later seen as a mandatory component for all future work to be done in Indonesia.

An Unexpected Hitch in the Educational Efforts

One of PATH's major claims to fame as an organization is its experience in creating culturally sensitive materials designed for illiterate and semiliterate audiences. The materials include brilliantly composed drawings that carry vital health information and a carefully crafted emotional message—as opposed to written texts that would be indecipherable to their target audience. Material was tested, pretested, and retested for the Indonesian project to make sure the immunization message would motivate action. Talented language experts, artists, and designers were used to mount this information and education campaign, which PATH felt was indispensable for an effective program.

In 1987, when one of the three district leaders in the province refused to allow the distribution of the hepatitis B manual, PATH's commitment to popular participation was put to the test. One memo noted:

I think we should be cautious in assuming that the Central Lombok Bupati [District Leader] and his wife have a monopoly on truth about what kinds of information will work best with their "subjects." While they may feel that commanding, rather than explaining in a comprehensible, culturally appropriate way, works best, [PATH] experience suggests otherwise.[127]

The Bupati had objected because the manual used the local language, Sasak, which was usually not written; thus there was a strong possibility that some words would be badly misinterpreted, radically changing the meaning of the text. (Apparently, since there is no standard Sasak lexicon, the original slogan prepared for the hepatitis campaign could be read as "Don't Immunize" your child.) At first the Task Force/PATH members were angry with the Bupati, but they came to recognize that he had correctly pinpointed a problem that the project teams had missed.[128]

PATH was willing to reconsider and rethink specific problems in its educational texts and to adjust them to local cultural and political realities, but it was loath to give up its general approach and the ideals behind it:

> At PATH we try to make pictorial materials as nearly "self-explanatory" as possible, but at the same time to make certain, through careful training, that the people using the support materials clearly understand the messages and explain them well. . . . [M]eanings are in people, not the pictures (or text.) That is why we test so carefully and keep our ears open for comments like those of the Bupati. . . . Of course . . . it is important to work with community leaders. . . . [However,] if villagers understand why they should do something . . . higher compliance will result. The "rulers" who do the motivating, and the motivated, [both] need support materials.[129]

PATH's long and successful experience in using print material as a way of contacting semiliterate people made its use an integral part of their commitment to popular participation. When a question was raised about "whether or not booklets are used by illiterates,"[130] it was not dismissed but was treated as "an empirical question to be investigated through an evaluation,"[131] though with the strong expectation from past PATH experience that the answer would be a reassuring yes.

Unfortunately, this was not the case in Lombok. As described by D'Agnes,

> In retrospect, we made the mistake of pre-selecting the media for our primary target audience, e.g., print media for parents, without first determining the reach of print . . . on Lombok and the communications preference of our . . . audiences. . . . [Rather,] if we had piloted a media reach and preference study first, we would have quickly learned that print media is not the preferred means by which Indonesians like to receive health or other information.[132]

This problem was compounded by the failure of the Provincial Team and the PKK to distribute the written material; in addition, transportation and geographic problems made it impractical for either the Ministry of Health or the PKK to maintain the distribution system. But the real problem was that the medium was wrong—PATH experience not-withstanding. A reliance on print material for parents would make the education program neither replicable nor sustainable in Lombok.

Disappointed, PATH's first response was to shift the use of the booklets away from parents and toward target hamlet leaders, their wives, and limited numbers of PKK cadres instead. Written materials were only used to motivate parents when they were directly applied by training monitors.

Still, PATH did not entirely give up trying to reach the mass audience directly, and it experimented with alternative media such as radio and mosque loudspeaker systems.[133] It found that television was a good medium for reaching the population because, despite the lack of widespread private ownership, large numbers of people had access to the sets that existed.[134]

For people who are experts on making every donor dollar count and minimizing wasted effort, the educational campaign, which involved a considerable expense, was a notable exception to the rule. In its proposal to USAID to continue its work in Lombok on a second project, PATH stated that while the Lombok project showed the necessity of working with and educating both local and national governments during every stage of the work, "participatory communication processes should always be an integral component of primary health care programs, particularly in programs using appropriate health technologies"[135] and the local language must be used. PATH made this argument despite the fact that the Lombok experience did not really support this position.[136] Here, PATH subordinated short-run cost savings in order to lay a foundation that it hoped would produce long-term sustainability.

As we will see in the next chapter, PATH and the Task Force found the situation in Thailand similar to that in Indonesia, despite the greater Thai literacy rate and familiarity with printed materials. PATH adjusted to the necessity of working with different leadership levels and emphasized their education, but it continued to prioritize mass education as being of vital importance. In both Thailand and Indonesia the brilliant print materials were often not distributed, usually not read, and rarely given much attention, even among vaccinators. Rather, leadership groups gave orders that infants should be immunized, and the people simply cooperated, despite the fuzzy ideas parents had about what was going on. Such procedures violated the PATH philosophy, but they worked.

Still, PATH also kept expanding its educational outreach efforts to the general population, despite their redundancy. D'Agnes clearly explains the motivation behind their dogged persistence:

The Government said you don't have to educate the mother [because] we will tell the leader to tell them. But we felt it is important to educate the mother. Tons of data show that what really impacts infant mortality is education at the level of the mother. We didn't want to just stick needles in arms. We want to do more. . . . [For example, the medical] structure that gives shots requires mothers to walk long distances [to the health center], one time a month. They must be motivated to do this. They have to give up one day's work in the fields. Even if the headman says come they don't always come. [It is a] very slow process to get them to realize they have the power to prevent death . . . [due to their religiously supported] fatalism. [People are] . . . very poorly educated. We feel what we do is a form of popular education. Yes, some will act on orders by the government [and] we have taken advantage of that. But we want to do more. It is a long process![137]

And they were willing to go the distance.

The Task Force and PATH personnel worked diligently to overcome the immediate obstacles, to find neglected opportunities, to simplify procedures, to correct mistakes, to do what had to be done to make the project work in Lombok, and to provide a usable model for the rest of Indonesia. When the Task Force and PATH found that administration and record keeping at the permanent health centers and the periodic outreach clinics were generating too many mistakes, they worked for simplification and integration of records. When they found that mothers did not understand the need for more than one shot of hepatitis B vaccine, they pushed for more education and worked to lessen the need for multiple contacts with the mothers by helping test multivalent vaccines (e.g., those combining hepatitis B and diphtheria antitoxin). They also tried to deal with the problems created by the high turnover of local medical staff, the continuous replacement of senior administrative staff, the movement of PKK members, and the powerful influence of traditional medicine practitioners.[138]

The outcome of their work was the definitive demonstration that hepatitis B vaccination could be successfully integrated into the EPI. Adding hepatitis B did not overburden the existing system—which was the initial fear of both UNICEF and WHO, the sponsors of the EPI— and it made the system more effective and increased overall coverage for the EPI vaccines. The reason for this was that, in order to get hepatitis B to infants within the first week of life, the Task Force had to help improve, simplify, and sometimes create a more efficient birth registration system. It was thus possible to find infants more easily and efficiently for the purpose of administering any vaccination. By educating mothers about the importance of early hepatitis B immunization and the need for all three shots, workers found they could educate them simultaneously about the EPI in general, so that enthusiasm created for hepatitis prevention carried over to other vaccinations. EPI coverage increased in the target areas and in the surrounding districts as well. The project also demonstrated that no significant difference in protection existed among children who received two rather than three doses of vaccine, which raised important possibilities for future campaigns.[139]

Nationwide Adoption of a Modified Immunization Program

The model program was so successful that the Indonesian government announced its intention to institute universal hepatitis B immunization throughout Indonesia starting in April 1991. The assumption was that if it worked in Lombok, it would work anywhere. This was a great triumph for the Task Force.

The pleasure of victory was, however, tempered by the government's announcement that it would not replicate the entire program—specifically, it would not follow through on the model project's commitment to give newborns the first shot in the home within seven days after birth. The government felt it was too expensive to bring the medical system down to the hamlet/home level. Since most Indonesian hepatitis B was transmitted horizontally from child to child, rather than from mother to child, they felt their position was medically as well as economically justifiable. The Indonesians also decided not to copy other aspects of the model project, including the birth notification system.

In the eyes of Brad Otto, the Task Force's representative in Lombok, this unfortunate decision resulted from powerful Indonesian attitudes that had resisted every effort to change. The issue of the replicability of the program had been given low priority compared with achieving high coverage in the core villages, regardless of the cost:

This shortsighted view only highlights the problem of "project mentality." Although the goal of the Model Project is to *integrate hepatitis B immunization into the routine immunization program.* Nothing about the activity has yet been considered *routine,* and those implementing the project fully expect to do so only as long as it is a "project." This is the overriding attitude expressed at the national, provincial, [and] district . . . levels.[140]

Despite unhappiness with the government's decision, D'Agnes felt that at some point the government would be willing to adopt the more effective early vaccination method and that it was correct in its assessment that the hamlet delivery system the Task Force had pioneered was not cost effective as long as only hepatitis B vaccine was in the payload. She regretted they had not realized this fact during the early years of the program, but she believed that the problem could be

rectified if a number of interventions were delivered together immediately after birth. This system would prove itself economical, even for
Indonesia.

When asked what he would have done differently if he could redo
the project, Widjaja said that he would have set up two different model
programs: one delivering the vaccine to newborns in the home during
the first seven days and the other using the existing village-level system, which provided vaccination in the second month. With the comparative data thus generated, differences in protection alone would
have persuaded the government to adopt the model project's methodology, regardless of the cost.[141] (It soon may be possible to compare the
results of the Lombok model with data from the rest of the country as it
adopts the village-level program, which initiates vaccination during the
second month after birth.)

At the end of the four-year hepatitis B model project, PATH (acting
independently of the Task Force) received funding for a child initiative
program that covered the same Lombok villages. This project built
directly upon the system created for hepatitis B vaccination; by emphasizing the ability of the health workers to deliver a number of vital
health services (from vitamin A supplements to tetanus shots), PATH
hoped to prove the desirability of extending the health system down to
the hamlet level.

From D'Agnes's viewpoint the hepatitis project had provided PATH
(and, indirectly, Indonesia itself) with a unique tool for improving
health throughout the country:

By the fourth year [of the program] we had a [de facto] "field laboratory" that
covers 1,000,000 people. We . . . h[ave] a laboratory to introduce modeling
[health] interventions: products, . . . educational messages, software/hardware.
[We can show] how they can be fit into the existing system. We have a site where
you can monitor, measure, assess . . . [and quickly] get feedback.[142]

D'Agnes believed the eighteen core villages of the hepatitis B project
could be used for intensive evaluation and that the rest of the Indonesian villages could be used to scale-up the interventions. The project
villages could be used to determine whether a health product is user-
friendly and, if it is not, to point up ways to refine it, thereby bypassing
many of the problems of "ivory tower" laboratory theorizing. The one
million people in the villages would produce enough data to convince
the government that something was doable, a conclusion which could
be easily dismissed if only the eighteen core villages were used. This
was an unexpected side effect of the hepatitis B program that nevertheless could potentially have a positive impact on the national hepatitis B campaign.[143]

Local Production of Vaccine

One of the other effects of the successful completion of the model program has been that it revived governmental interest in fostering local hepatitis B vaccine production. PATH originally became involved with hepatitis over the question of helping transfer vaccine technology to Indonesia. The transfer had been incorporated as one of the Task Force's major goals, though it was clearly recognized that it might be the hardest to achieve because of the politics of local production. PATH had found significant delays were the norm in Indonesia because of the many powerful groups that must be involved in such ventures.

PATH's belief that local vaccine production in Indonesia would be slow in coming was well founded. In addition, however, the Task Force itself had subordinated that goal in favor of creating the model vaccination program and lowering the price of the vaccine. One of the main effects of radically lowering the price of the vaccine on the world market would be to make local production less important, at least from an economic standpoint.

The issue recently resurfaced, however, as a number of politically powerful groups in the government became interested—chief among them was the Indonesian Ministry of Science and Technology. The Ministry saw the new national hepatitis program as being capable of generating a large market for a locally produced vaccine. (During the years of the model project, BioFarma, which had been initially intimidated by the idea of producing hepatitis B vaccine, had been reorganized under a more efficient and aggressive leadership which felt capable of entering the field.) The Minister of Science and Technology's primary interest was not to prevent the disease itself, but to use hepatitis B vaccine as a vehicle for propelling Indonesia into high technology. Thus he was interested not in producing a plasma-derived vaccine but rather in manufacturing a genetically engineered recombinant DNA vaccine. The Minister of Health, unlike the Minister of Science and Technology, continued to favor the local production of the simpler plasma-derived vaccine, which would be cheaper to manufacture and was within the technological reach of a developing country.

Key members of the Task Force, including James Maynard and Alfred Prince, continued to be strong supporters of the idea that Third World nations can and should produce their own hepatitis B vaccines. They saw the issue not purely as a matter of cost-accounting economics, but rather as one of national pride, which to them was a legitimate interest. However, while they believed that developing countries like Indonesia could safely produce high-quality plasma vaccines, they did not believe these nations could produce safe recombinant DNA vaccines. Infrastructure and quality controls can be put in place for the former, but not for the latter. This has put the Task Force and PATH in a difficult position. They want to assist Indonesia, but they do not want to help produce a disaster. D'Agnes's view of the situation perhaps most closely reflects the way the Task Force will handle this tricky subject: avoid getting into the middle of this potent political struggle at all cost, but if asked, help Indonesia produce the safest possible vaccine regardless of which type they choose. In present-day Indonesia, the Minister of Science and Technology appears to be better connected politically than does the Minister of Health. Ultimately, the comparative power of the rival Ministers and Ministries will determine which vaccine will be produced.

The likely producer of the new hepatitis B vaccine will be the state pharmaceutical company, BioFarma, the selection of which may also signal a major political conflict. There are at least some who believe that the choice of the newly upgraded public sector agency reflects a shift away from the private sector companies, represented by Kalona and Lembong, and the "unofficial" desire to promote ethnic Indonesian interests over those of the Chinese businessmen who have traditionally controlled the pharmaceutical industry.

Lack of Corruption in the Model Project

One of the most interesting aspects of the hepatitis B pilot program was the lack of corruption that characterized its execution. Since academicians frequently emphasize the centrality of corruption in Indonesian society, this finding is surprising. There were a number of reasons for this, foremost among them being the wholehearted support the program received from key government officials. The Governor of Lombok supported the fight against hepatitis B from the start and was willing to monitor the progress of the program even though it involved the lower levels of the hierarchy—a highly unusual state of affairs. Apart from any practical effects his intervention may have had, it had a great symbolic effect on his subordinates. The Minister of Health was also deeply committed, and as a result there was no need to provide incentive payments to individuals in the Ministry of Health to get things done. Incentives were used only when the Task Force and PATH needed the cooperation of officials outside the health ministry (e.g., those who controlled taxation of imported products, including vaccines, or the issuance of work permits for expatriates).[144] Even in these cases nothing more was required than "the [traditional] giving of gratuities [which were] . . . always necessary with low paid officials in the developing world,"[145] payments which do not merit the term "corruption." Finally, the program had the high-profile backing of President Suharto.[146]

On the local level there was no corruption or siphoning off of vaccine or syringes for the private marketplace because the program was seen as village- and people-oriented, with firmly based community support. It was not seen as an impersonal foreign program that could be "ripped off" without guilt.[147]

In addition, PATH's staff set up a system of checks that gave them more control over the situation than they had had in other programs. They did not supply the vaccine all at once; rather, they only provided enough for three months, and they carefully monitored how fast this amount was utilized. They knew how many syringes should be required to do the job, and they allowed only a fixed number for normal breakage. Later, they also regularly checked the stocks inventoried in the warehouse. Thus the program was kept corruption-free as a result of community ownership, national and provincial political support, and careful planning. Whether these checks on corruption will operate during the national program remains to be seen.

The Indonesian Model as a Prototype for the Developing World

The Task Force's work in Indonesia was a major success. Its accomplishments were many and of great importance for Indonesia and for the Third World as a whole. The model program broke the price of the hepatitis B vaccine: The pledge from Samsung/Cheil to sell the vaccine at $1 a dose in the public sector moved the question of hepatitis B vaccination from a low-priority issue to center stage in the world health community. At the same time all pharmaceutical companies were pressured into rethinking their marketing strategies. By having an international bid and tender that was won by the KGCC, the Task Force proved that the $1-a-dose goal was not simply a humanitarian gesture or loss leader but rather a viable economic possibility. Its model program in Lombok demonstrated that hepatitis B could be successfully integrated into the EPI without overburdening it. Indeed, addition of hepatitis B vaccine could help support and strengthen the EPI. The Task Force and PATH demonstrated techniques for bringing vaccination into the home immediately after a child's birth, even in the most inhospitable terrain. They showed that even poor Third World countries could establish mass immunization programs, and thus the foundation was laid for the eradication of both hepatitis B and the liver cancer that so frequently follows.

The Task Force's work in Indonesia also demonstrated the fundamental importance of cultural sensitivity when operating in the developing world. On countless occasions the model project would have failed if the foreign team had not been able to adjust to the political and social realities of Indonesia. It was vital for them to win over local and national business and political leaders, a task which could only be accomplished once they gained an intimate knowledge of and respect for the rules and etiquette of the society. Thus if the Indonesians did not want negative information communicated in the public eye, it had to be done in private—without witnesses. When it was discovered that local inhabitants would cooperate only after a direct command from someone high up in the hierarchy, then such an official had to be found. If local business leaders could only succeed as clients of powerful bureaucrats, then it was necessary to find the best politically connected entrepreneur with whom to work.

The group also learned that conditions in the field rarely conformed to experts' and informants' predictions. A successful project required constant adjustment to the physical, social, and political situations existing on the ground. Constant improvisation was necessary, whether it meant dealing with villages divided by an unbridgeable chasm, vaccinators who did not vaccinate, or a women's organization that existed only on paper. Rigid adherence to preexisting plans simply would not work.

The Task Force and PATH showed that by working within the system, they could help the Indonesians themselves reveal unexpected signs of flexibility, as long as their sense of propriety was not trampled on. These lessons served the Task Force and PATH well when they established model programs in other developing countries.

In December 1991 a final review meeting for the Lombok model project was convened, which provided the statistics that proved the program was a true success. In Indonesia, where 10 percent of the adult population are chronic carriers of the virus, more than 500,000 children born each year will join that group. Of that cohort 100,000–125,000 ultimately will die from cirrhosis or cancer of the liver. The results of the Lombok immunization project, if extended to the rest of Indonesia, would prevent 400,000 of those chronic infections and 100,000 premature deaths per year. Children who received all three doses of the vaccine and the first dose within seven days of birth experienced an approximate 80 percent reduction in carriership.[148] The public health benefits of this protection are magnified because child carriers are highly infectious and the new noncarriers cannot spread the disease to their neighbors. The birth notification system established by the program revealed that more than 80 percent of births in the project area were recorded, where previously official birth certificates were completed in less than 4 percent of the cases. Before the project started fully 55 percent of the children between the ages of 1 and 2 had no contact with the EPI, and only 15 percent were fully immunized with the EPI vaccines. After four years of the project, more than 90 percent of the children in the core villages were fully immunized. In addition, the success of the Lombok model program provided a strong incentive for the government to establish a nationwide hepatitis B immunization program, just as the Task Force had hoped.

A Possibly Destructive Conflict over the Task Force's Relationship to PATH

Along with all their successes, the Task Force experienced one troubling internal conflict during the course of its Indonesian work. The Task Force's effectiveness, in Indonesia and elsewhere, had been significantly enhanced by its association with the PATH organization. Without the expertise, skillful preparation, and constant vigilance of PATH-Seattle and the continuous on-the-ground presence and cultural/political sensitivity of PATH-Jakarta (and PATH-Bangkok), the Task Force could not have succeeded. However, even under the best of circumstances, when leadership groups meet only periodically and are served by permanent secretariats (as is the case, e.g., for the World Health Assembly of WHO and the WHO apparatus), they run the risk of finding themselves upstaged by their servants. When, as in this case, the bureaucracy (i.e., PATH) is a separate, independent organization, the situation is exacerbated, especially since the Task Force's secretariat was the driving force in the creation of the dominant organization in the first place. In this situation the key question becomes, "Who is the dog and who is the tail?" Many of the Task Force members were very sensitive to this problem; the most outspoken of them was Gust.

During the first formal meeting of the newly created Task Force in Nairobi, Kenya, in March 1987, the issue of the group's relationship to PATH created a "very traumatic" situation.[149] As far as Gust was concerned, Richard Mahoney seemed to envision the group's members as being PATH-like employees, though only of the part-time variety. But Task Force members were not willing simply to be consultants to PATH.[150] The roles had to be reversed.[151]

PATH accepted the legitimacy of the Gust grievance. As a result a document was prepared that stated explicitly that the Task Force had chosen PATH to work with it, and that the group could dismiss PATH in the future if it saw fit. In addition, in an attempt at intraorganizational unity, James Maynard, who was retiring from the CDC, was appointed a vice-president of PATH so that he could act as a bridge between the two organizations. His special status was symbolized by the fact that both boards had the power to fire him.[152]

But once Maynard was located within PATH-Seattle, the question of where his ultimate loyalties lay became an issue. In addition, since Maynard and Mahoney worked full-time on Task Force business and were in daily contact with the Chairman, Alfred Prince, decisions were often made by that triumvirate, without the consultation of the entire membership. There was a feeling that the advantages of speed and efficiency provided by the leadership acting on its own came at too high a price. In an attempt to counter this problem, Maynard was given responsibility for issuing a monthly newsletter. Such detail work, however, was not his strong suit, and the newsletter came out only sporadically, thereby further exacerbating the problem.[153] As late as 1990, in response to what was still seen as an unresolved problem, Gust wrote to Mahoney:

We need to clarify the relationship between PATH—acting as PATH, PATH acting as a WHO Collaborating Centre and PATH acting for the Task Force. All the existing Task Force [TF] members have expressed concern about this area and it was also noticed by outside observers. . . . In the past two years, TF members have sometimes felt that the roles have been reversed, with decisions being made or initiated in Seattle, and then the TF being asked to approve them . . . often retrospectively. . . . I think that PATH needs to help to promote the TF as an entity. . . . [I]n Lombok Brad [Otto] is seen as a PATH (not TF) employee, both projects in Asia are widely perceived as PATH projects. Your own paper at the Houston [Task Force] meeting was under the name PATH![154]

Gust was quite right about how the Task Force was perceived. Key people in Indonesia and Thailand saw the Task Force as simply an arm of PATH—a misperception that was further supported by Task Force members' frequent use of PATH stationery when communicating with Indonesian officials and the even more frequent use of the phrase "PATH wants" in written documents where the phrase "the Task Force wants" would have been more appropriate. The fact that PATH offices in each country were very active in implementing Task Force policies and that the whole issue of hepatitis B had been a PATH concern for years inevitably made the Task Force seem to be the servant, not the master, in the relationship. Insofar as PATH had created goodwill or valuable connections in Thailand and Indonesia, the confusion helped the Task Force; insofar as PATH had made enemies and aroused jealousies, the confusion hindered the Task Force. This is not to say that the two organizations were seen as entirely identical. The Task Force membership's high prestige did not go unnoticed, and it clearly eclipsed that of PATH and its employees. Maynard, Prince, and Gust carried weight that PATH could never exercise on its own, and yet the Task Force's aura of independent authority was surely compromised.

The conflict over primacy between the Task Force and PATH was a major irritant for years; nevertheless, what is most significant about the conflict is not that it existed, but that the various parties were able to accept the tension and still maintain the vital relationship between the organizations. In most such situations this kind of disagreement would have led to either internal or external collapse. But the Task Force members and the leadership of PATH were able ultimately to subordinate their personal and institutional egos to the common goal. This, more than anything else, has been the hallmark of the Task Force-PATH collaboration. When push came to shove the need for cooperation in the successful fight against hepatitis B and liver cancer took precedence over the internal organizational battles.

Notes

1. The existence of a new manufacturer in Singapore threatened the very possibility of establishing local hepatitis B vaccine production in Indonesia. Many of the nations of Southeast Asia (as part of the Association of Southeast Asian Nations) had signed an agreement to share a variety of facilities as a way of controlling expenses while still meeting area-wide needs. The idea was that each country would be given the sole right to manufacture a specific product and then be allowed to export it to the others, thus avoiding needless duplication. Since Singapore was planning to produce hepatitis B vaccine, it appeared Indonesia might be barred from entering the field. However, the Singapore company faced a number of significant problems that clouded its future. For example, while it needed to import infected plasma from Indonesia or Thailand, it was illegal to export blood from the former, and the latter had contracted to ship its blood to Holland for processing into vaccine. Ultimately, the President and Minister of Health of Indonesia decided that the country was not bound by the original agreement and could produce hepatitis B vaccine if it wanted to (memo from Anton Widjaya to Leona D'Agnes, October 26, 1985, concerning a meeting of the Indonesian National Hepatitis Functional Group).

2. Lucien W. Pye, *Asian Power and Politics: The Cultural Dimensions of Authority* (Cambridge, Mass.: Harvard University Press, 1985), 116.

3. Ibid.

4. Ibid., 306.

5. Ibid.

6. Ibid.

7. Ibid., 307–308.

8. Ibid., 309.

9. Ibid., 301.

10. Ibid., 119.

11. Ibid.

12. "Drs." refers to a Dutch degree, "Doctorandus," and is roughly equivalent to a Master's degree.

13. Memo by Leona D'Agnes to Hepatitis B File, dated May 27, 1985; memo by Carl McEvoy to Hepatitis B File, July 17, 1985.

14. Memo by McEvoy to Hepatitis B File, July 17, 1985. There was a belief at this point in time that recombinant DNA production was much simpler and easier to carry out than plasma-derived vaccine production. Such was not the case, however.

15. Memo by D'Agnes to Mahoney, August 17, 1985.

16. Memo by D'Agnes to Mahoney, May 27, 1985.

17. Memo by D'Agnes to Mahoney, August 17, 1985.

18. Memo by Mahoney dated October 9, 1985, about a conversation with D'Agnes on October 2, 1985.

19. Letter from PATH (with no signature) October 17, 1985, addressed to Dr. Marisi Sihombing, Advisor to the Minister of Health.

20. As we saw in Chapter 2, when the Minister of Health went on a PATH-sponsored trip to the East Coast of the United States, Mahoney had trouble with a businessman who was part of the group. That man was Lembong, and they got into a verbal skirmish over whether Mahoney should accompany them on a side trip to Merck headquarters. After that trip Mahoney wrote D'Agnes that Lembong's behavior made future cooperation with him impossible, which was a loss, since there was the possibility of a fruitful venture with him on oral rehydration therapy (memo by Mahoney to Hepatitis B File, May 12, 1986).

21. Memo by Henry Wilde to Mahoney, January 22, 1986.

22. Memo by D'Agnes to Hepatitis B File, April 24, 1986.

23. Memo by D'Agnes to Gordon Perkin, April 13, 1989, about PVO (Office of Private and Voluntary Cooperation); Jonathan A. Green, "Report to PATH Re Health Link Project: Subproject Review, January and February 1986," addressed to USAID. In an interview on June 21, 1991, Green said, "The head of the section of USAID–Bureau of Private Enterprise, couldn't come to grips with the fact that PATH wasn't primarily private sector. She was a Reagan person. This was before the Reagan Revolution was finished. She had to deal with quasi-public firms. She couldn't deal with the fact that PATH was non-profit."

24. Memo by D'Agnes to Hepatitis B File, April 24, 1986.

25. Memo by Mahoney to Indonesian File, May 17, 1985.

26. Memo by Wilde to Mahoney, June 24, 1985.

27. Memo by Carl McEvoy to Hepatitis B File, July 17, 1985; Lembong said that the "committee on hepatitis that PATH has heard about is not a formal group but a list of interested individuals which will be brought together to get an informal consensus on the problem."

28. Memo by D'Agnes to Mahoney, August 17, 1985.

29. This is Wilde's comment about BioFarma's attitude after meeting with members of the staff, but it is information that Kalona would have as well (memo by Wilde to Mahoney, #4, December 19, 1985).

30. Memo by Mahoney to Shin Seung-il, December 2, 1985.

31. Memo by Mahoney to Hepatitis B File, Asian Trip Report #5, February 18, 1986.

32. Interview with Anton Widjaya, January 19, 1992.

33. Memo by Wilde to Mahoney, #4, December 19, 1985.

34. Memo by D'Agnes to Mahoney, March 14, 1986; memo by Mahoney to Hepatitis B File, #4, February 20, 1986.

35. Memo by D'Agnes to Mahoney, May 16, 1986; May 29, 1986.

36. Memo by D'Agnes to Mahoney, May 16, 1986.

37. Memo dated May 6, 1986, dealing with the meeting among Cheil, P. T. Wigo, and PATH.

38. Ibid.

39. In the initial discussion with Kalona, Widjaya had commented that any vaccine production project would probably have a high degree of government interference in it, but he did not feel that the government would try to exclude the private sector—any such beliefs were misinformed. He felt that the government would only try to exclude the private sector from vaccines already being produced or tested in government facilities (memo by Wilde to Mahoney, #2, June 24, 1985).

40. Interview with Widjaya, January 21, 1992.

41. PATH, "Health Link Six-Month Report Covering the Period September 1984–February 28, 1985" (1985). Hepatitis B vaccine was on the list of areas of interest but not near the top.

42. Interview with D'Agnes, January 21, 1992.

43. Memo by Mahoney to Hepatitis B File, May 17, 1985, reporting on a May 2, 1985, meeting with Kalona. Mahoney's description of Widjaya is consistent with his not knowing that he is a PATH consultant.

44. Interview with D'Agnes, January 2, 1992.

45. Memo by D'Agnes to Mahoney, May 20, 1987, regarding pre-project activities related to the model immunization project. The importance of Widjaya's role became very clear on one of the few occasions that he was unable to carry it out. As a result of conflicts between the National and Provincial Hepatitis Teams concerning the model demonstration project, the Minister of Health wrote a strongly worded letter to PATH and the Task Force saying that all activities (including provincial work) had to be channeled through the Ministry (in Jakarta) and that the National and Provincial Teams, not PATH, had to take the active role. This type of statement, which restricted PATH and the Task Force's freedom of action and communication, was exactly what they wanted Widjaya to help avoid.

46. Interview with D'Agnes, June 27, 1991.

47. Interview with Maynard, June 25, 1991.

48. Interview with Widjaya, January 21, 1992.

49. Interview with Gust, February 24, 1991.

50. Interview with D'Agnes, January 21, 1992.

51. Memo by Mahoney to Hepatitis B File, November 15, 1985, concerning the meeting with Maynard.

52. Memo by Wilde to Mahoney, #8, December 26, 1985, concerning November 26, 1985, meeting. Adhyatma's attitude ultimately changed, and he became a major supporter of the hepatitis B project. He ultimately became Minister of Health. He was so supportive that D'Agnes has no memory of there ever being any opposition from him about giving hepatitis B a high priority (interview with D'Agnes, January 21, 1992).

53. Karl Jackson, "Bureaucratic Polity: A Theoretical Framework for the Analysis of Power and Communications in Indonesia," in *Political Power and Communications in Indonesia,* edited by Karl Jackson and Lucian Pye (Berkeley, Calif.: University of California Press, 1980), 17.

54. Memo by Wilde to Mahoney, #8, December 26, 1985.

55. Memo by Mahoney to Hepatitis B File, #12, September 30, 1985, concerning the meeting with Fakhry Assaad of WHO and Maynard of the

Centers for Disease Control. D'Agnes does not take credit for originating the model idea concept, probably because it was just one of many ideas she generated at the time. At this point her main focus was local vaccine production, and a model program would have been used to further that goal. When the Task Force actually adopted the idea, it increasingly replaced the goal of local vaccine production, which required some time for adjustment by the local PATH office (interview with D'Agnes, January 21, 1992).

56. Memo by Mahoney to Hepatitis B File, #12, September 30, 1985, concerning the meeting with Fakhry Assaad of WHO and Maynard of CDC.

57. Interview with Maynard, July 7, 1993. Maynard's and Shaw's travel expenses were paid for by PATH, not the U.S. government.

58. Letter from Shin Seung-il to the Task Force, August 15, 1986.

59. Interview with D'Agnes, January 21, 1992.

60. It was at this meeting in March 1987 that all the members of the expanded Task Force came together and it took its final, fully mature organizational form, with elected officials and formal structure. To Maynard the "real" Task Force only came into existence when the group met and constituted itself as an entity; everything before that date was only a proto-Task Force (interview with Maynard, July 6, 1993). Given the tensions which, as we will see, exist between the full Task Force and its secretariat, PATH, such a view must be politically appealing to many on the Task Force, but I think it is stretching reality to divide the group's history at the Nairobi Conference. Clearly the Task Force existed when Mahoney, Maynard, and Prince created it, and it expanded when they decided to expand its membership; no new group came into existence in Nairobi.

61. Memo by Mahoney to D'Agnes, April 3, 1987.

62. Ibid.

63. Letter from Shin Seung-il to Dian Woodle of PATH, July 24, 1987.

64. International Task Force on Hepatitis B Immunization, "Task Force on Hepatitis B Immunization: Preliminary Criteria for Selection of Vaccine for the Indonesian Model Immunization Program," 1987.

65. Interview with Gust, February 24, 1991.

66. Memo by Mahoney to Dian Woodle of PATH, July 23, 1987. Confirmation of KGCC's willingness to supply vaccine to others at the same price came on July 24, 1987, in a letter from C. H. Kim of KGCC.

67. Memo by Shin to Dian Woodle of PATH, July 27, 1987.

68. Memo by Mahoney to Shin, July 29, 1987.

69. Interview with Prince, January 29, 1991.

70. Interview with Nancy Muller of PATH-Seattle, June 27, 1991.

71. Memo by Mahoney to Dian Woodle of PATH, July 10, 1987.

72. Memo by C. H. Kim of KGCC to Dian Woodle of PATH, July 24, 1987.

73. Interview with Gust, February 24, 1991.

74. Interview with Maynard, June 19, 1991.

75. In a letter to Dr. John Sever of Rotary International (September 11, 1987) requesting support for the Thai Model Program, Maynard wrote: "We believe that if one takes a realistic view, the Lombok project is by no means assured of success. . . . The Thai project, on the other hand, provides an opportunity to study the integration of hepatitis B vaccine into EPI under much more favorable conditions."

76. Letter from Mahoney to William Muraskin, August 20, 1992.

77. Interview with D'Agnes, June 27, 1991.

78. International Task Force on Hepatitis B Immunization and PATH, "A Model Immunization Program for Hepatitis B in Lombok, Indonesia: Protocol" (1987), 1.

79. Ibid., 3.

80. Ibid., 4.

81. Ibid., 5.

82. Ibid.

83. Ibid., 6.

84. Ibid., 6–7.

85. Ibid., 8.

86. Ibid., 9.

87. Ibid.

88. Ibid., 10.

89. Ibid., 11, 15.

90. Ibid., 16.

91. Ibid., 12.

92. Ibid.

93. Interview with D'Agnes, June 27, 1991.

94. Ibid. Widjaya said that government red tape in Thailand and Indonesia makes it almost impossible to try to get something done (memo by Mongkil Chayasirisobhon of PATH to Mahoney, August 6, 1985).

95. Ibid.

96. Interview with D'Agnes, June 27, 1991.

97. "A Model Immunization Program," 13, 14.

98. Interview with D'Agnes, June 27, 1991.

99. Ibid.

100. Interview with Otto, June 27, 1991.

101. Interview with D'Agnes, January 21, 1992.

102. Ibid.

103. Memo by Scott Wittet of PATH to D'Agnes, February 17, 1987.

104. Memo by D'Agnes to Scott Wittet of PATH, March 13, 1987.

105. Ian Gust, "Public Health Control of HBV: Worldwide HBV Vaccination Programme," in *The Hepatitis Delta Virus*, edited by John L. Gerin, Robert Purcell, and Mario Rizzetto (New York: Wiley-Liss, 1991), 333–342.

106. Scott Wittet, Anne Peniston, and Holly Blanchard of PATH to Hepatitis B File, "Feedback from Field on Project Protocol Issues," July 9, 1987.

107. Ibid.

108. Ibid.

109. Ibid.

110. Ibid.

111. Ibid.

112. Thomas R. D'Agnes, Draft Report, "Assessment of Training Needs, Resources and Capabilities in Lombok, N.T.B. for the Model Immunization Program for Hepatitis Vaccine," 1987.

113. Interview with Leona D'Agnes, June 27, 1991.

114. Interview with Otto, June 27, 1991.

115. Ibid.

116. Ibid.

117. Interview with D'Agnes, January 21, 1992.

118. Interview with Otto, June 27, 1991.

119. Interview with D'Agnes, January 21, 1992.

120. Ibid.

121. Memo by D'Agnes to Nancy Muller of PATH-Seattle, January 16, 1990, in which she talks of the need to help parents in Lombok who do not understand the need for the complete series of vaccine shots: "To enhance parental understanding . . . several social marketing and social advertising activities will be undertaken. . . . For example, social marketing approaches will be used to give value [to] . . . exclusive breast feeding. . . . Similarly, social advertising techniques will be applied to market the concept of complete immunization . . . using Islamic NGOs [non governmental organizations] and verses from the Koran to instill the concept of parental responsibility for childhood immunization."

122. Interview with Otto, June 27, 1991.

123. The Office of Communicable Diseases, NTB Province, Indonesia, and PATH, Jakarta and Seattle, "Beliefs and Practices Regarding Illness and Immunization in Lombok as Perceived by Village Parents, A Summary of Findings" (1987).

124. Ibid.

125. Interview with Otto, June 27, 1991.

126. Interview with Nancy Muller of PATH-Seattle, June 25, 1991.

127. Memo by Scott Wittet of PATH to Chris Ajamiseba, November 13, 1987.

128. Interview with Otto, June 27, 1991.

129. Memo by Scott Wittet of PATH to Chris Ajamiseba, November 13, 1987.

130. Ibid.

131. Ibid.

132. Memo by D'Agnes to Maynard, June 2, 1989.

133. Ibid.

134. Interview with D'Agnes, January 21, 1992.

135. Letter from Gordon Perkin, President of PATH, to Sally H. Montgomery, Deputy Assistant Administrator, PVO Child Survival Grants Program, Office of Private and Voluntary Cooperation, Bureau for Food for Peace and Voluntary Assistance, dated January 18, 1990.

136. Ibid.

137. Interview with D'Agnes, January 21, 1992.

138. Letter from Dr. Tilman Ruff (a colleague of Gust) to D'Agnes, November 15, 1989, including a copy of an article entitled "Integration of Hepatitis B Immunization in Lombok (Indonesia)," by Tilman Ruff, Ian Gust, Augustine Sutanto, James Maynard, Antonius Widjaya, and Soedarto Sosroamidjojo.

139. Draft of the "Minutes of the Annual Meeting of the International Task Force on Hepatitis B Immunization," Houston, Texas, April 3–4, 1990. However, Mark Kane felt that WHO would never recommend two doses (rather than three) because of its preference for a "simplify, simplify" approach.

140. Memo by Otto to Hepatitis B File, August 4, 1990. Italics in original. Otto mellowed on this criticism by the time he was interviewed on June 27, 1991, when he said, "I think they are justified in not replicating the reporting system—not enough resources. Do it slowly, after they know local conditions."

141. Interview with Widjaya, January 21, 1992.

142. Interview with D'Agnes, January 21, 1992.

143. Ibid.

144. Interview with Widjaya, January 21, 1992.

145. Written comment by Prince to William Muraskin, August 1992.

146. Interview with D'Agnes, January 21, 1992.

147. Ibid.

148. "Lombok Model Hepatitis B Immunization Project Final Review Meeting, Lombok, December 5–6, 1991." Those who received fewer than three shots, or the first shot more than a week after birth, also had a substantial reduction, but more in the 60 percent+ range.

149. Interview with Gust, February 24, 1991.

150. Interview with Maynard, June 1, 1991.

151. Interview with Gust, February 24, 1991. In a letter from Mahoney to Gordon Perkin, President of PATH, dated September 9, 1986, he said it was not reasonable for the New York Blood Center to be a member of the Task Force due to its Cheil association and thus "The Task Force would be shown to be an activity of PATH."

152. Interview with Maynard, May 1, 1991.

153. Report by Maynard (to Task Force Members), June 4, 1990.

154. Letter from Gust to Mahoney, April 24, 1990.

Chapter 4
The Task Force in Thailand

For the International Task Force on Hepatitis B Immunization to prove that large-scale hepatitis B immunization was a realistic goal for the developing world, a number of successful model programs had to be established. The logical site for a second project was the Kingdom of Thailand. Thailand, like Indonesia, had a significant hepatitis B problem, a large population, and an already existing governmental concern with the disease. In many ways Thailand presented a better opportunity for the Task Force than Indonesia had because the former was more economically and socially developed, had a higher rate of literacy, a booming economy, and a growing number of skilled scientists and technicians. As in Indonesia, the Task Force had the benefit of a Program for Appropriate Technology in Health (PATH) office and PATH experience in dealing with key people in the government and in the universities.

However, the situation in Thailand would prove to be far more complex and difficult than in Indonesia because the Task Force decided not to subordinate its efforts to transfer vaccine technology to the job of creating a model immunization project. Instead, it pursued both goals simultaneously. As a result the Task Force became more deeply immersed in the scientific and governmental politics of Thailand than it had been in Indonesia, and the Task Force's activities were even more directly affected by PATH's earlier in-country involvement.

The Thai venture demonstrated both the advantages the Task Force and PATH workers had when operating in the developing world—resulting from their cultural sensitivity and political savvy—and the pitfalls lurking in the convoluted sociopolitical environment of Thailand. The Task Force was to achieve a major victory in Thailand (the agreement of the government to institute a nationwide immunization program) but also suffer its greatest defeat (the collapse of its efforts to transfer hepatitis B vaccine technology). To make matters worse, the complexities of the Thai technology transfer issue fostered serious disagreements within the Task Force which threatened its cohesiveness, if not its very existence. Once again, its ability to weather such disputes resulted from the membership's willingness to subordinate ego and personal philosophy to achieving the overarching goal.

The problems the Task Force faced in Thailand derived from the large number of competing economic groups and individuals in the country. The Thai economy was expanding rapidly as it strove to emulate the Pacific Rim nations and become a modern industrial state. The result was the proliferation of many competing groups of individuals with entrepreneurial and scientific ambitions, all jockeying for position in the coming new order. These rival groups were unequally connected to the ruling bureaucracy. For the Task Force to succeed it had to assess the scientific and business acumen of the various individuals and also the degree of political influence each possessed. As we will see, the Task Force received considerable help from knowledgeable local sources in judging the attributes of the different parties, and it was very successful in many of its assessments. However, in one key instance—its choice of the Thai Red Cross to receive the transfer of vaccine technology—the Task Force was inadequately informed regarding the quality of the organization's political connections. That failure ultimately led to the Task Force's failure in establishing local hepatitis B vaccine production in Thailand.

PATH in Thailand Before the Task Force: Rabies and Hepatitis B Vaccine Production

To understand the Task Force's activities in Thailand, we must first look at the role PATH played in the years before the Task Force was formed. PATH had become aware of the local hepatitis B problem in 1984 as a by-product of its inquiries into the feasibility of transferring advanced rabies vaccine to Thailand. At that time, the Thais manufactured a rabies vaccine that was substandard by international criteria and which put the patient at significant risk of a severe reaction. The Thais were aware of the problem and unhappy with it.[1] A number of different groups of scientists, centered in the universities and in the Thai Red Cross, were interested in producing a safer and more modern rabies vaccine. The ambitions of these individuals reflected the growing desire of Thai scientists and institutions to make Thailand one of the leading modern economies of Asia, as well as to increase their own power and prestige while bettering their personal financial situations. Many of the scientists/academics had visions of developing income-producing entrepreneurial ventures of the type pioneered by their counterparts in the United States.

For almost all of these groups, production of rabies vaccine was seen as intimately linked with the manufacture of hepatitis B vaccine. Their reasoning was that a rabies vaccine production plant would require facilities and staff that could also be used to make hepatitis B vaccine. "Piggybacking" hepatitis B vaccine production onto the rabies vaccine industry was needed to make the latter economically viable, because the potential market for rabies vaccine was quite limited compared with that for hepatitis B. As a result, most PATH inquiries about rabies vaccine ended up with a discussion of hepatitis B vaccine production.

The most important scientific groups in Thailand were associated with either Chulalongkorn University or Mahidol University in Bangkok. Many ambitious projects, all requiring outside help, were discussed there. The academic promoters were linked, or implied they were linked, to important people in the government or private enterprise.

Thailand, like Indonesia, has been characterized as a bureaucratic polity, where little gets accomplished without government approval, often manifested through the direct involvement (and profit) of senior bureaucrats. The Thai government, even more than that of Indonesia, has in recent years given its blessings to dynamic entrepreneurship as a means of developing and strengthening the country, while simultaneously enhancing bureaucratic rule through the flow of increased profits.[2]

PATH found academics who wished to engage in vaccine production everywhere in Bangkok. One prominent individual, Dr. Prasert Thongcharoen, Chairman of the Department of Microbiology, Siriraj Hospital Faculty of Medicine, told Richard Mahoney he was "moving rapidly forward"[3] in creating a new company to produce biologics, and was hoping to produce animal and human rabies vaccines as well as vaccines for hepatitis B and Japanese encephalitis. He also claimed that the Crown Properties Company, one of the groups from which the royal family obtained a portion of its income, would be one of the investors in his new enterprise.[4] In addition, Dr. Amorn Nondasute, Permanent Undersecretary of Health, was interested in a hepatitis B program and had asked Dr. Prasert to help carry it out. On another occasion, Mahoney met with Dr. Kachorn Pranich, former Chairman of the Department of Microbiology of Chulalongkorn University, who strongly praised the plans for hepatitis B vaccine production coming out of the Thai Red Cross Institute. The school's Department of Microbiology was closely associated with the Red Cross Institute (which was located on the Chulalongkorn University campus), and the Thai Red Cross, significantly, was under royal sponsorship, with the Crown Princess[5] an active patron and protector.

The Red Cross Institute of which Kachorn[6] was so supportive was one of the divisions of the Red Cross Society and had many important Chulalongkorn professors associated with it: Dr. Visith Sitprija (Vice Dean of the University), Dr. Praphan Phanuphak, and Dr. Supawat Chutiwongse (Chairman of the Department of Obstetrics and Gynecology), of Chulalongkorn University Hospital, were among the most prominent and active. When Richard Mahoney met with Visith and Praphan, he was told that they also represented a group of academics and public sector individuals interested in setting up a company to make both hepatitis and rabies vaccines. They informed him that the Thai Red Cross was already involved in an arrangement with the Dutch Red Cross to ship Thai blood plasma (contaminated with hepatitis B virus) to the Netherlands, where it would be processed and returned as finished vaccine. However, this arrangement did not allow the Thais to develop their own expertise in manufacturing the vaccine. Praphan, who did his Ph.D. work at the University of Colorado, believed he could transfer the hepatitis B technology from the professors he worked under there, while the technology for rabies vaccine could be obtained from the Wistar Institute in Philadelphia.

Mahoney was attracted to Visith and Praphan's plans but had to point out that since PATH's Health Link program was funded by the Bureau of Private Enterprise of the U.S. Agency for International Development (USAID), which only allowed them to assist private companies, PATH could not directly aid the Red Cross Institute. (As we have already seen, this exclusive focus on the private sector was a constant irritant for PATH in Southeast Asia, since it was based on the false assumption that a clear-cut division existed between the private and public sectors.)[7] Praphan and Visith responded that their group would like to form a private company but they lacked the professional business expertise required. However, they knew of a well-connected physician,[8] the "son of a multi-millionaire," who recently had equipped a new military hospital established by an important senior Thai general—in other words, a politically well-placed individual in a country where connections are indispensable. A few days later they arranged a meeting with the physician-entrepreneur who said he was willing to work with both the University and the Red Cross—though, confidentially speaking, he was willing to do it alone, since as a private company he could work faster.

The Small Margin of Separation Between Private and Public Sectors

For Mahoney, having a private businessman interested was a positive development, but he felt that maintaining a good relationship with the public sector, represented by Drs. Visith, Praphan, Kachorn, and Supa-wat, was also quite vital. He would not go forward with a prefeasibility study without their express approval.[9] At a later meeting with Visith, Mahoney said that he had met with their entrepreneurial friend and discussed a prefeasibility study for both hepatitis B and rabies vaccines. However, PATH considered it premature to become involved with only one company. Rather, it wanted the professors who were associated with the Red Cross Institute (i.e., Visith and co-workers) to help carry out the studies.

Mahoney believed that it was crucial to continue to involve Visith and his colleagues at each step of the process, from prefeasibility study through actual implementation.[10] Success in Thailand required main-taining a fine balance between the public and private sectors, and undercutting the former for the latter, in keeping with Washington's unrealistic preference, was to be carefully avoided. Since Mahoney felt that PATH had a special role to play in working to encourage private companies to serve the public interest, he did not see the two sectors in opposition to each other. In this respect his view was similar to the one held by the Rockefeller Foundation, which had been seriously consid-ering ways in which the public sector could encourage the private sector to produce vaccines while fostering cooperation between the erstwhile rivals.[11]

When Visith and Praphan invited Mahoney to an important business dinner to discuss the feasibility study for producing hepatitis B and rabies vaccines, he was forced to reveal a further limitation on his free-dom of action. The Bureau of Private Enterprise mandated not only that PATH deal with private companies but that PATH be reimbursed for their feasibility studies expenses. Thus, according to Mahoney,

I explained that the Bureau . . . expected us to generate income and that our success would be measured, in part, on the extent to which we did receive reimbursement for expenses incurred. . . . [This was to explain] why we are operating in certain ways, i.e., more as a commercial, industrial firm than as an international nonprofit, foundation-type agency.[12]

To get around this requirement, Mahoney suggested that PATH itself do a prefeasibility study of the two vaccines, thus eliminating the need for fees.

This situation, like the one in Indonesia, created embarrassment for Mahoney and severely damaged PATH's reputation in Thailand for years to come. Even after PATH had located funders that did not burden it with such counterproductive requirements, the suspicion of profit-making self-interest clung to the group. No matter how politely Mahoney's Thai listeners may have reacted to his explanations, lingering doubts were left that would be later reinforced when PATH, acting as the Task Force's secretariat, championed the Cheil vaccine as the best solution to the technology transfer problem.

As Mahoney continued to pursue the twin problems of hepatitis and rabies, he and his staff had to maneuver very carefully and discreetly around the rivalries, personality conflicts, and status struggles that permeated the Thai government and industry. For example, when PATH worked to bring the Thai Red Cross together with the Mérieux Institute of France (initially to supply the most advanced form of rabies vaccine and ultimately to transfer the technology for locally producing it), Mahoney was warned that the French company was "uneasy with the idea that PATH was the star of the show."[13] It was suggested that the situation could be defused if those involved emphasized that the Thai Red Cross was the primary agent, only drawing upon PATH assistance as needed.[14] PATH members tried to accommodate to the situation by severely lowering their profile, but their defensive maneuver did not succeed in defusing the competition. When the final agreements were negotiated, Mérieux managed to exclude PATH from the arrangement entirely. Since PATH staffers were new to the game of vaccine technology transfer, they did not recognize their vulnerability in the face of the more sophisticated Mérieux lawyers and staff.[15] They had to lick their wounds and look upon their loss as a learning experience.

Maneuvering Carefully Through Local Institutional and Personal Rivalries

As Mahoney continued to deal with the leaders of the Red Cross Institute he noticed that at least one key person was unhappy with the developing situation:

I have felt concern for some time that Dr. Praphan does not see us as someone who is helping him, or the Red Cross Institute. To the contrary, I think that Dr. Praphan [as Scientific Director of the Thai Red Cross] sees us as a group that is not as technically qualified as he is, but yet seems to be making decisions with which he does not always agree. Other people in the Red Cross Institute listen to our advice, and this is a loss of face [for him]. . . . Should we invite him to be involved as a principal investigator in one or more of our projects?[16]

The alienation of an important leader of the Institute over a question of status was a danger that had to be carefully avoided.

While PATH was deeply involved in wooing individuals in the Red Cross Institute and increasingly successful in convincing them of the importance and utility of setting up a cooperative venture with the private sector, the question still remained as to "whether they [could] convince the administrative, old guard of the Thai Red Cross parent organization of this."[17] In the eyes of some, the Red Cross was just "awakening from a 30 year slumber,"[18] and its ability to be flexible was open to doubt.

In addition, the fact that the Red Cross Institute and the National Blood Center, another division of the Red Cross Society, were major institutional rivals, with conflicting goals but overlapping interests, did not bode well. When it came to hepatitis B vaccine production, the National Blood Center, not the Institute, owned the blood (which constituted the raw material for the vaccine) and would have the ultimate decision-making power, regardless of the Institute's opinion. PATH had good relations with the leaders of the Blood Center, including its Director, Dr. Chaivej Nichprayoon, but not quite as close as those it had with the Institute's staff.

In an attempt to investigate all existing resources for vaccine development, PATH staffers met with the powerful and prestigious Dr. Natth Bhamarapravati, President of Mahidol University. Natth was a dynamic administrator and internationally respected scientist who had developed one of the Dengue fever vaccines. Unfortunately, Mahidol University maintained a long-standing rivalry with Chulalongkorn University and its Red Cross Institute. If one of the Institute's advantages was royal patronage and the favorable interest of the Crown Princess, the Mahidol Foundation could make a similar claim, as could Natth himself. Natth was the driving force behind the creation of a new giant campus for his university at Salaya, outside Bangkok, and he was interested in fostering PATH's involvement there. Trying to utilize the resources of both Mahidol and Chulalongkorn Universities placed PATH in the middle of a difficult political situation. At least initially, however, there was little choice.

President Natth was a very influential and knowledgeable figure who appeared to be the key person in Thailand on the subject of the hepatitis B vaccine.[19] He was also well connected with high government officials. He told Henry Wilde (an advisor to PATH in Thailand) that the Ministry of Health, in collaboration with Mahidol University, was planning a pilot study of hepatitis B vaccination of newborns in an as-yet unspecified location. He told Wilde that the entire question of large-scale administration of hepatitis B vaccine was a "very politically sensitive"[20] one in Thailand.

Wilde found Natth to be well informed regarding the different types of hepatitis B vaccine. When Wilde told him that PATH was interested in transfer of technology and was enthusiastically negotiating with Merck to obtain their new recombinant DNA vaccine, Natth expressed a marked skepticism about the venture. In his opinion the recombinant

DNA vaccine derived from yeast (which Merck was pioneering) was a passing technology whose methods were complicated and costs much too high. In addition, it required costly equipment such as fermentation tanks that could not be used for anything other than yeast production. He went so far as to speculate that its weaknesses were exactly why Merck was so interested in transferring the technology. In Natth's opinion, the future belonged to mammalian cell–derived DNA vaccines.[21] He was skeptical of all companies interested in transferring technology: no manufacturers transferred successful products, only unsuccessful ones.[22]

Despite these views, Natth was optimistic about the future for science in Thailand because of the abundance of well-educated and creative Thais in technical fields and the quality and quantity of research being done there. Such talented people needed only small grants to steer them into areas that would be commercially and practically exploitable. When Wilde asked him if PATH could help form a private company to assist such individuals, Natth said steps in that direction had already been taken by a number of scientists, but he had slowed them down because the basic research and development had not yet progressed far enough. PATH could indeed help, but sometime in the future.[23]

Natth's persuasive arguments regarding the yeast-derived DNA vaccine was one of the factors that convinced Wilde that PATH should stop investing money in the yeast-derived–technology transfer.[24] While Mahoney ultimately came around to Wilde and Natth's point of view, he was slower to change. Mahoney felt that the DNA possibility should be kept alive because senior officials in both Indonesia and Thailand were clearly interested in it, as were the four major vaccine companies that were working on hepatitis B vaccines. In addition, he had been assured by internationally reputable scientists that the recombinant DNA production was indeed simpler than the plasma-derived vaccine process.[25] Mahoney also believed that Thai bureaucratic politics and rivalries might be unduly influencing President Natth's position.[26] In Thailand one always had to be aware of the possibility that political infighting rather than objective observation shaped the advice one received. But while such caution could be wise under some circumstances, it could also delay the acceptance of accurate information.

President Natth was also openly skeptical of the desirability of the transfer of plasma-derived hepatitis B vaccine technology. He saw it, too, as a transitory technology and believed there was little reason to invest in it. Small-scale production by the Thai and Dutch Red Crosses was reasonable, but he would not push for such a venture at Mahidol University—at least not until someone showed production could be done successfully.[27] Opposition to plasma-derived vaccine, along with other factors, would ultimately turn PATH and the Task Force away from Mahidol University and toward the Thai Red Cross.[28]

Vaccine Production Is Not Separable from Mass Immunization Campaigns

While PATH's pre–Task Force interest in hepatitis B in Thailand was primarily concerned with fostering local production of the vaccine, increasing evidence showed that production could not be looked at in isolation. Dr. Supawat, Director of the Red Cross Institute, made this point quite strongly in a meeting with PATH's local representative, Mongkol Chayasirisobhon. Supawat related the details of a meeting at which James Maynard of the Centers for Disease Control (CDC) had been involved. Maynard had asked about the possibility of plasma-derived vaccine production in Thailand. Supawat had told him that the key problem was not production per se, but rather whether the Thai government would adopt a policy favoring the establishment of a nationwide immunization program. This was the fundamental question to be answered before one worried about producing vaccine. When Maynard went on to ask if the Dutch Red Cross (which had agreed to import Thai blood and process it into vaccine) would transfer the vaccine-making technology, Supawat again told him that this was not the crucial question. The establishment of a national policy committed to mass immunization had to take priority. Supawat went on to tell Mongkol that once the question of hepatitis B vaccine production became relevant, it was important that it not be purely a Red Cross project but that it also involve the Ministry of Public Health and related organizations, such as the Government Pharmaceutical Organization (GPO). Since high-level policy questions had to be answered before production would be put on the agenda, Supawat saw no immediate role for PATH.[29] (Later, after Mahoney and Maynard met, it was Maynard who acted as the spokesman for establishing a model immunization project as the first step toward any effort to transfer vaccine technology.)[30]

Meanwhile, talk was increasing in government circles about beginning some sort of immunization program. The Ministry of Public Health's Hepatitis Control Committee began to consider establishing a program for vaccinating all mothers who tested positive for hepatitis B e antigen (i.e., the carrier most likely to be infectious).[31] Within a few months, the Institute's Praphan was told that the Ministry had indeed decided to begin such a program. This commitment meant that 30,000–40,000 infants would be vaccinated, requiring 90,000–

120,000 doses of vaccine. Thus hepatitis vaccine was finally becoming a very hot topic in Thai government circles.[32]

The Role of the Dutch Red Cross

The initial effect of this heating up of the hepatitis B issue was that the key people at the Thai Red Cross Institute, among them Drs. Supawat and Praphan, became interested in expanding the fledgling agreement negotiated with the Dutch Red Cross. The two sister Red Crosses had set up an arrangement in which the Thais sent hepatitis B carrier blood to the Netherlands, where it was processed and returned to Thailand as finished vaccine. Since the two Red Crosses had already established a mechanism for providing vaccine for blood, it was hoped that they could quickly increase the supply. In addition, the Dutch would be the logical choice to ultimately supply the technology and know-how for establishing local production. Since the Thai Red Cross did not have the staff to do the manufacturing alone, a private enterprise partner would eventually be needed. PATH could play a role in negotiating that issue, as well as in helping the Thais and the Dutch to carry out their work.[33]

The increased Thai interest in the Dutch connection was potentially a positive event in the fight against hepatitis B in Thailand, though it was not perceived that way by PATH. The Dutch Red Cross was seen more as a competitor than as a potential collaborator. Seen objectively, the issue as to whether the Dutch or PATH helped the Thais achieve hepatitis B vaccine production did not matter, because PATH's goal would be accomplished either way. Indeed, the likelihood existed that PATH could use its resources to facilitate the Dutch-Thai activities. But the underside of PATH's dynamism and ambition to do good was its tendency toward organizational imperialism: It wanted to be the best, to be the leader, to be at the center of things. While the PATH membership understood that success in the developing world often required keeping a low profile, giving credit to others for one's own achievements, and following a policy of self-abnegation (a policy it followed most of the time), it nevertheless found it hard to do so consistently. It especially did not like to be left out of the action. PATH had a strong sense of mission; but a sense of mission and a seat on the sidelines did not go well together. As Mahoney put it:

[O]ur . . . "success" with rabies will make people very sensitive to our probing around in hepatitis B. Nevertheless, . . . we should move aggressively, since it seems that there is a real opportunity to work here, to make a real contribution . . . [but there are forces that] could result in projects being completed . . . without our involvement. I believe the reason we must be involved is because we can assure that, to the extent that private-sector groups are involved, attention is paid to the needs of the public sector and alternatively, that to the extent the public-sector organizations are undertaking the project, they use the highest-quality methodologies and management approaches which are usually found in the private sector.[34]

Mahoney felt that PATH had to stop approaching hepatitis B in Thailand as an outside observer and become an integral player. This sentiment was reinforced by the fact that PATH had, by late 1985, determined that the New York Blood Center (NYBC)/Cheil vaccine and process were superior to what the Dutch had to offer. As a result, Mahoney did not look favorably upon the Red Cross development; instead, he wanted to take the "leadership role in the hepatitis B technology transfer issue."[35]

In this instance, being aggressive meant intervening directly within the Red Cross Institute. Dr. Praphan had become a key supporter of the Dutch connection. He had visited the Netherlands a number of times and was impressed with what he saw there. Yet Mahoney felt that Praphan could not fully understand the Dutch situation vis-à-vis other producers from his brief visits to the Netherlands, and therefore recommended that PATH go over Praphan's head and speak directly to Drs. Supawat and Visith to see whether the Thais would be interested in a collaboration with the Samsung group (the owners of Cheil).[36]

Henry Wilde, PATH's chief consultant in Thailand, was closely involved with the Red Cross Institute and knew how disastrous such a confrontational course of action would be. Wilde quickly responded that Praphan had positive feelings toward PATH which he had been nurturing for a long time. In addition, Praphan was both an important scientist and a personal friend. It made no sense to go over his head on this issue. The Dutch and the Thais had begun their collaboration before PATH's entrance on the scene. The Dutch vaccine was not only half the cost of Merck's, but a good one at that. According to Wilde, the Thais would need private sector involvement when they moved to the manufacturing stage, and that would be the time for PATH to get involved. To interfere earlier by "lobbying against the Dutch [would] impair PATH credibility"[37] and accomplish nothing. In Wilde's view, the two Red Crosses were tied together by good relations not only between their staffs but also between their respective royal patrons. PATH could conceivably go around the Thai Red Cross and look for another firm to use the NYBC/Cheil technology, but this would offend its outside critics as well as the Red Cross. Thus there was no choice for PATH but to be an observer rather than a major player, for the time being.[38]

Wilde's reasonable advice probably helped prevent a serious blunder that would have severely compromised PATH's (and later the Task

Force's) future effectiveness. As it turned out, however, Wilde had overestimated the sense of loyalty the Thai Red Cross felt toward the Dutch Red Cross. Their goal, like PATH's, was to get a cheap vaccine and to obtain the technology to produce it locally. Loyalty to a sister Red Cross was of secondary importance to that objective. When a better option appeared they were quite willing to take it—though preferably in a way that was not harmful to the other party.

Although PATH, as a result, took a far less aggressive stance toward the Dutch than had first been contemplated, it did not sit inactively on the sidelines or accept Wilde's assessment that there was little role for it at present. PATH continued to press the advantages of the Cheil vaccine and the NYBC methodology on the Thais, to work to maximize competition between the drug companies (using each pharmaceutical company's most recent lowest bid as a weapon to force down the price of its rivals), and to bring Thai and Indonesian groups together with Cheil to work out limited agreements on hepatitis diagnostics—and, it was hoped, to lay the foundation for future local vaccine production. PATH did all this without direct confrontation, alienation of allies, or blatant undercutting of long-established cooperative relationships. Indeed, PATH was so effective that when Wilde later met with Dr. W. G. Van Aken of the Dutch Red Cross, Van Aken could good-naturedly say that he held no grudge against PATH for "'mucking around in the hepatitis vaccine business in Asia, and for having started a small price war.'"[39] Van Aken said he too would like to see a vaccine cheap enough that mass immunization campaigns would become practical.

Political and Technological Factors Favoring PATH over the Dutch Red Cross

Over time, the increasingly fluid vaccine situation in Thailand favored PATH's position, independent of its own actions. Many Thais, both inside and outside the Red Cross, came to appreciate that there were many options for procuring and producing hepatitis vaccine. The Dutch provided one possibility, but their vaccine had significant drawbacks. Important people in the Ministry of Health were very unhappy with the fact that the Dutch vaccine did not meet the biological standards for hepatitis B vaccines of the World Health Organization (WHO) and thus lacked its "stamp of approval."[40] In addition, it became clear that the Dutch Red Cross's production technology was inefficient and outmoded, especially in comparison to the Cheil/NYBC process. (Even the Dutch were painfully aware of this fact; they had begun discussions with the NYBC to cooperate in upgrading the Dutch technique.)

The key problem with the whole idea of local hepatitis B vaccine production or the establishment of a national immunization campaign remained that the vaccine was still too expensive. The Dutch vaccine, while relatively cheap, was not cheap enough to solve the cost problem. Furthermore, other pressing disease problems in Thailand—including an increase in incidence of malaria and Japanese encephalitis and weaknesses in the diphtheria-pertussis-tetanus, polio, and measles eradication programs—continued to take precedence over hepatitis B.[41] These diseases would continue to hold sway until someone dramatically lowered the price of vaccine and simultaneously made a compelling argument for pushing hepatitis B to the top of the priority list. PATH, rather than the more sedate Dutch Red Cross, was the group actively working on the issues of both price and urgency.

While the Dutch Red Cross was interested in playing a more significant role in Thailand and Indonesia, providing a less expensive vaccine, and transferring technology, they had certain handicaps which PATH did not share: They lacked the resources to support staff members in those countries for the extended intervals that would be required for them to establish themselves and their projects. In addition, they lacked "the ability to overcome the many political . . . obstacles that one would have to expect to face in a developing country."[42]

In Indonesia, for example, they had been approached repeatedly by people interested in establishing a vaccine arrangement, including Dr. Masri Ruslam, Director of the Indonesian Red Cross. Masri wanted to set up an agreement similar to the Dutch-Thai blood-for-vaccine exchange. The negotiations initially looked promising, but then the Minister of Health unexpectedly blocked the agreement, citing the Indonesian law that forbade the exportation of domestic blood. Van Aken felt this was simply a political ploy since the problem could have been easily resolved: "someone must have lubricated the gears quite well in Indonesia, and . . . this lubrication was not in our favor."[43] The nonprofit Indonesian Red Cross (like the Dutch Red Cross) was not well versed in political machinations, and the Dutch decided to drop the issue "unless they [were to be] approached from Indonesia by someone who is able and willing to manipulate the political zig-zags which would have to be overcome."[44]

Van Aken was correct: the Dutch Red Cross did not know the right people in the government. Its contacts were limited to the Indonesian Red Cross, and within the competitive client-patron system that organization was simply not well connected enough to achieve an agreement.[45] Lack of local, politically astute representatives hampered the Dutch in both Indonesia and Thailand.

Increasingly, even key supporters of the Dutch connection within the Thai Red Cross were willing to look elsewhere, though they wished to do so in a way that would not create bad feelings.[46] Certainly PATH's championing of Cheil was an important ingredient in their change of mind, but the Thais made it clear that they still had doubts about the Koreans and would, if given the choice, choose an established manufacturer such as Pasteur Vaccins over Cheil—even if they had to pay slightly more for the vaccine. To go with Cheil (or the Dutch for that matter) the Thais would have to be offered a major price discount.[47]

Pasteur Vaccins was becoming more competitive as a result of the pressure exerted by PATH.[48] At one point it appeared to be willing to go as low as $2 a dose for the vaccine—which, if true, would have beaten not only the Dutch but even Cheil's price at the time. The offer turned out to be illegitimate (it came from a Taiwanese company that had received its technology from Pasteur only on the condition that it not sell vaccine outside the country), but PATH was able to use it as a weapon in its campaign to force Cheil to lower its price. In a meeting between Cheil and the Thais, with Wilde present, the Koreans were pressured into agreeing to match Pasteur's price, whatever it might be.[49] The Thai representatives made it clear that the Ministry of Public Health would not be interested in establishing a mass hepatitis B campaign unless the vaccine price fell to at least $2 per infant dose.[50] (At this point the Cheil agent suggested that Wilde and Praphan go to Seoul and "present the case for a mass market vaccine to his superiors"[51] since headquarters' thinking was still focused on a narrower market. Later, as we have seen, Cheil went down to $1 a dose, but not as a result of the pressure from Thailand.)

The Dutch Red Cross Unexpectedly Withdraws from the Vaccine Competition

Ultimately, the Dutch Red Cross hepatitis B vaccine ceased to be a factor in Thailand, not because of PATH's promotion of Cheil or Pasteur's increased competitiveness, but because the Dutch simply withdrew from the hepatitis vaccine production arena entirely. The main cause of their withdrawal, however, lay outside of Southeast Asia.

The Dutch had realized for some time that their manufacturing process was inefficient. They had good relations with the NYBC, which, like itself and the Thai Red Cross, was a non-profit organization. There was also a significant personal link between the groups since Alfred Prince's heat-inactivation technology was actually a refinement and improvement of the method the Dutch had originally pioneered. As a result of these connections, they started to negotiate an agreement with the NYBC to collaborate on upgrading their methods.

The Dutch looked forward to the possibility that they and the NYBC might combine their work and achieve an inexpensive, second-generation, plasma-derived vaccine designed for the developing world. Dr. A. W. Reesink of the Dutch Red Cross was especially concerned that the two groups avoid competing or engaging in the slanderous campaigns that had become the custom among the larger manufacturers. In speaking to Wilde, Reesink said that

> the battle between Pasteur and MSD [Merck], in particular, has hurt the hepatitis vaccine issue since it has resulted in the introduction of unnecessary and counterproductive regulatory efforts by WHO that have been used to keep out competitors. We all . . . concluded that our efforts should be directed not in producing another competitive high-or-middle priced vaccine for the middle classes who do not really need the vaccination.[52]

Instead, they were to develop a "poor man's" vaccine.

For at least some PATH employees such a prospect was very exciting. Wilde, who was always less committed to Cheil than others were, believed the situation was very favorable:

> If our objective is to bring a good inexpensive hepvac [hepatitis vaccine] to Thailand, it matters little if this is done by the NYBC-Cheil group, Pasteur, MSD [Merck Sharp and Dohme] (who do not seem very interested) or the NRC [Netherlands Red Cross].[53]

PATH's role would come into play in setting up the commercial part of the venture.[54]

Prince and the NYBC were also enthusiastic about the Dutch plan because a modified Dutch vaccine would in fact be a second version of the Prince vaccine, and the Dutch could be licensed to sell it in areas of the developing world, such as Latin America, which the Cheil-NYBC agreement did not include. Indeed, there was a possibility that the Dutch Red Cross would be included as a member of the still-forming Task Force.[55] (When Wilde told the Thais that a Task Force had been formed, he included the Dutch Red Cross as part of it.)

Mahoney, once again demonstrating his basic flexibility, began to appreciate the possible benefits of speeding up the transfer of vaccine production technology to Thailand by using the Dutch Red Cross rather than the Cheil Sugar company once the Dutch switched to the NYBC methodology. PATH could work to facilitate the process,[56] thus meetings were arranged to solidify the relationship between the Dutch and the New York group.[57] Because the Dutch Red Cross did not receive government subsidies and had to pay its own way, the transfer of technology would require outside financial help. Mahoney quickly offered PATH's aid in preparing a feasibility study for the proposed transfer.[58]

Unfortunately, while negotiating to improve their vaccine, the Dutch manufactured two bad batches that produced low titers of antibodies in recipients. Some of the ineffective lots of vaccine were used in the Netherlands and others were shipped to Thailand, creating both a health problem and a public relations nightmare. The Red Cross made public announcements encouraging people to come in for booster shots. Initially, they felt they could solve the problem and would continue to sell the vaccine.[59]

Around this time, the Dutch informed the Thais that they were interested in transferring their entire hepatitis B vaccine production plant to Thailand. The heads of the National Blood Center of the Thai Red Cross were very excited about the Dutch offer. However, Drs. Supawat and Praphan of the Red Cross Institute (which often competed with the National Blood Center) saw the offer as downright dangerous. They said the technology was just too complex, and by the time it was set up other manufacturers would capture the market.[60] Wilde, on the other hand, felt there were advantages in such a transfer, including the enhancement of Thai national pride and conservation of scarce foreign exchange. In addition, a plant jointly operated by the Dutch and Thai Red Crosses could export some of the vaccine back to the Netherlands, thus helping to finance the venture at the same time it increased the prestige accruing to Thailand. Wilde admitted there were drawbacks as well, since the price they charged would have to be higher than a large manufacturer such as Pasteur could offer. In addition, Wilde noted, the established companies could fight the Thai vaccine

[by starting] a slander campaign and indirect efforts through their well established channels to government decision makers. . . . [Also, there is a] long standing competition and jealousy between the Medical Science Division of the Ministry of Health, the Government Pharmaceutical Organization, and the Thai Red Cross. This might hinder such a project which requires cooperation with the Ministry, the ultimate user of the vaccine.[61]

Already the larger manufacturers were actively publicizing the latest Dutch problems and spreading the false rumor that the Dutch Food and Drug Administration had withdrawn its approval of the vaccine.[62]

The Dutch became more and more discouraged about their hepatitis B vaccine production. The unfavorable publicity surrounding the bad vaccine lots was traumatic for them and had damaged their reputation. The fact that WHO's requirements kept their vaccine (both old and new) from meeting WHO standards also embarrassed the Dutch and made them all the more eager to get out of production. Adopting the Prince/NYBC methodology would be expensive and time-consuming, and the new Merck recombinant DNA vaccine had just been approved by the Dutch government for sale in the Netherlands. All of these developments were disheartening. The Task Force became concerned that the Dutch would simply drop the hepatitis B vaccine, which was what their increasing pessimism suggested.[63]

The Dutch incentives to stay in the field and help transfer hepatitis B vaccine production technology were also undermined by their growing doubts that the Thais would successfully receive it. Prof. Van Aken felt that both the Thai and Indonesian Red Crosses had underestimated the complexities involved in producing a viable vaccine.

[The Dutch Red Cross feels that] producing a safe and effective vaccine is a complicated, time-consuming venture which requires the full attention of the scientists and technicians involved and has no room for amateurs. Performing good quality control and safety tests at the end may well be the most difficult [part of the] process. . . . Dr. Van Aken has not been convinced that the organization required to do this type of thing presently exists in Thailand and Indonesia. . . . They are aware . . . that most of the people who have the technical and theoretical background to do this type of work have many other chores to do and simply cannot devote themselves . . . to doing a good job in plasma processing or vaccine development.[64]

Wilde suggested to Van Aken that bringing in a private company as a partner for the Thai Red Cross would solve this problem, but the fears of failure persisted.

In the end, the Dutch Red Cross did in fact leave the field in 1987, thereby nullifying their offer to transfer hepatitis B vaccine technology. (Significantly, Mr. Arie Langstraat of the Dutch Red Cross called upon Wilde of PATH to inquire how best to approach the Thai Red Cross so as to end their hepatitis B vaccine relationship without endangering their general relationship.)[65] Thus the disappearance of the Dutch competition, which a year earlier would have been viewed as a purely positive event by PATH, had been transformed into a loss and a gain for it and for the International Task Force on Hepatitis B Immunization that had recently come into existence.[66]

The Dutch withdrawal radically changed the technology transfer situation in Thailand. Although PATH had some regrets over losing the Dutch Red Cross as a potential partner, there was great excitement that the Task Force and PATH now had a golden opportunity to operate unimpeded in Thailand. They could now redouble their energies in championing Cheil as the most appropriate source for both vaccine and vaccine technology.[67]

The Major International Vaccine Companies
Meet the Task Force in Thailand

Just at the point that the negative publicity surrounding the Dutch vaccine was at its height (late 1986), a major scientific meeting, the First International Conference on the Impact of Viral Diseases on the Development of Asian Countries, was convened in Bangkok. The conference was a significant event for the new Task Force, and it was well represented there. The meeting provided an occasion for Task Force members to build bonds among themselves and to meet with key people from the Thai Red Cross as well as with important Thai decision-makers such as President Natth and Dr. Prasert. The conference also gave Task Force representatives international exposure by allowing them to meet with United Nations and WHO officials. An all-day sight-seeing trip provided the opportunity for members of the Task Force to meet with Dr. Umenai Takusai, head of Viral Disease at the Western Pacific Region Office of WHO, and with Dr. Yuri Ghendon of WHO-Geneva. Maynard was able to use this time to explain their position at great length.[68] The conference also provided the occasion for Task Force members to interact with the most powerful commercial drug companies and to present the Task Force as a group to be reckoned with.

It appeared to the Task Force members that the meeting was dominated by the large pharmaceutical companies (SmithKline, Pasteur Vaccins, and Behring/Hoechst), which set the agenda and paid the bills. As far as the Task Force was concerned, the companies used the conference simply as a forum to argue over who had the best vaccine and the product most likely to succeed in the marketplace. Pasteur aggressively pushed its plasma-derived vaccine and contended that heat-inactivated vaccines (i.e., the Cheil and Dutch vaccines) were of poor quality and questionable safety. The other companies piped in with the same theme. Wilde was particularly angered by what he saw as the commercialism of the meeting and the "obvious efforts of manipulating the program on the part of the three large sponsors"[69] to exclude competitors such as Cheil. PATH tried to get Prince or Shin Seung-il onto the program but was foiled. Finally, Wilde managed to get Shin on the platform, though only as a replacement speaker.

The Task Force members felt that the drug companies responded to Shin's presentation in a hostile manner. There were two SmithKline-sponsored scientists who spoke; as far as PATH observers were concerned, they did little more than monopolize the question and answer period. They asked nitpicking technical and statistical questions, apparently for the primary purpose of preventing any substantive discussion of the merits of the Cheil vaccine or the charges made against its production methodology.[70]

Maynard was the only Task Force member able to get the floor and attempt to rebut the charges that the heat-inactivation process was unsafe and inefficient. Audience members apparently were annoyed enough at the large companies' obstructionist tactics that they gave Maynard a round of applause after he spoke.[71]

Donald Douglas, one of PATH's local representatives in Thailand, felt that SmithKline's attack on Shin may have helped more than it hurt because it was so heavy-handed and intemperate that it made Cheil look like an Asian underdog, unfairly attacked by large multinational companies. Their behavior also made transparent "[their] attempt . . . to control and guide . . . [a] supposedly scientific meeting for commercial purposes,"[72] which was very off-putting.

Despite the clear hostility the large manufacturers displayed toward the Cheil and Dutch vaccines, their attitude toward the Task Force and PATH was considerably more ambivalent. They feared the Task Force would create a price war at their expense and push them out of their markets, but they were nevertheless anxious to be part of any successful projects the Task Force might undertake. Pasteur's attitude was representative. As Wilde saw it:

> It is quite obvious that the Pasteur group is deeply troubled by the activities of the Task Force . . . [and] troubled by the high likelihood that the Task Force will succeed in raising . . . money which will then be used for two or three large EPI [Expanded Programme for Immunization] pilot programs. They can see themselves being put into a position where they will have to lower the price to cost or less in order to retain the private market. . . . [T]hey [however] made it . . . clear that . . . they would like to negotiate with the Task Force and be asked to participate preferably as a sole supplier . . . for these pilot programs.[73]

Pasteur was willing to negotiate the price, perhaps going as low as $3–4 per adult dose, depending on the packaging.[74]

SmithKline (Belgium) also met privately with the Task Force and asked to be included as a supplier for future large-scale public-sector vaccine purchases. Like Pasteur, SmithKline was willing to negotiate on price but wanted the Task Force to stop promoting the $1-a-dose figure because it was creating public expectations and pressure on the companies to meet that price. SmithKline was, however, unofficially willing to endorse the $1 price as an ultimate goal.[75] At the same time, Pasteur met with the PATH people and discussed both past and future collaborations with them, as they attempted to obtain more information on the Task Force and its objectives.

The net effect of the Task Force's appearance at the conference was to demonstrate that the subject of hepatitis B vaccine pricing was going to be an area of continued conflict and hostility. Nevertheless, a significant new player existed that had to be taken seriously and negotiated with, even while established players tried to beat back its direct challenge.

The events of the conference foreshadowed the Task Force's future influence in the hepatitis B field, but they also raised some powerful fears among Wilde and Donald Douglas, PATH's two main representatives in Thailand. They had intimate knowledge about the Thais' sentiments, and they feared that the Task Force and PATH, in their enthusiasm, were unaware of what was going on locally. Douglas succinctly expressed both his and Wilde's view:

PATH and the Task Force still face an image of too-close association with Cheil. This could hurt us with key Asian decision makers . . . because of our previous work promoting transfer of Cheil technology to Thailand and Indonesia before the Task Force was conceived. The . . . insistence on $1.00 per dose is another reason we are linked to Cheil. . . . We risk raising unattainable expectations with the . . . price.[76]

Both Douglas and Wilde felt that establishing the independent credentials of the Task Force was of vital importance, and the best way to do that was to take seriously "Pasteur's suggestion of working with several companies in the field trial stage"[77] rather than just Cheil. At this time (December 1986) neither PATH headquarters nor the Task Force was particularly sympathetic to these kinds of suggestions.

Obtaining Support for a Thai Model Hepatitis B Program

Pasteur and SmithKline's belief that the Task Force was actively interested in moving ahead with a number of national model projects was, of course, correct. In Thailand the key job for the Task Force was to reach out to various parts of the government bureaucracy and make the case for a pilot project. Individuals and groups interested in such a program already existed, but they needed help to become an effective force. For example, at the Virus Conference Maynard met with President Natth, who expressed strong support for a demonstration project in Thailand. He said that government planning on such a project had already begun, and he offered to intervene with the top Thai governmental panels at the appropriate time. In fact, he told Maynard, he was a member of the National Thai Task Force on Hepatitis Containment, appointed by the Ministry of Public Health, which would be the key body that would make recommendations to the government.[78]

To get things moving Douglas and Wilde invited members of the Thai Hepatitis Action Group to a meeting. Present at the gathering were Dr. Supawat of the Red Cross Institute; Prof. Chaivej, Director of the Thai Red Cross Blood Bank; Dr. Praphan; Dr. Supamit Chunsuttiwat, representing the Ministry of Public Health; and Dr. Sompon,[79] a member of the Ramathibodi Hospital Staff and an influential Thai Senator. The Thais were already aware that the Task Force was actively planning a project in Indonesia, and the purpose of the meeting was to inform the Thais that the Task Force was interested in stimulating and sponsoring projects in Thailand as well.

The members of the Thai Hepatitis Action Group were also members of the important National Thai Task Force on Hepatitis Containment, which advised the Ministry of Health. Dr. Supawat opened the discussion by saying that the group should come up with suggestions and perhaps a plan to entice the Task Force to get involved. After much discussion some key conclusions were reached. First, several well-placed members of the decision-making staff of the Ministry of Public Health who were interested in hepatitis prevention had to be reassured that after the pilot project was over the work would continue, and that the price of the vaccine would be low enough to permit a sustained effort. Second, any initiative should originate from the existing National Task Force Committee, many of whose members were present at the meeting. The initiative might involve a pilot project in one or two provinces and should concentrate on identifying practical problems of logistics, distribution, and administration of hepatitis B vaccination, as well as evaluation of the effects of the vaccine. Dr. Supamit, the representative of the Ministry of Public Health, was encouraged to prepare a preliminary plan and to check to see whether such a design already existed at Dr. Natth's Mahidol University.

Douglas of PATH would simultaneously prepare a document outlining ways in which the Task Force might be enticed into helping execute such a project. Supamit's and Douglas's plans were to be presented by a suitable person, such as Dr. Sompon, to the Ministry of Public Health, as well as to other government and Royal Court officials. The group reacted favorably to the Dutch Red Cross offer to transfer vaccine technology to Thailand, which was seen as a way of making the activities begun by the pilot project sustainable after it ended. All agreed that the transfer would work only if the Dutch were willing to continue their involvement after local production was established.

At the end of the meeting it was decided that further discussions should take place between Supamit and his superiors at the Ministry of Public Health to explore the political and bureaucratic implications of their plan. Supawat and others would talk with Sompon, who had good connections with the Ministry, the legislative branch of the government, and the Royal Court. Most of those present felt that the Minister himself should not be approached until there was some consensus among the lower-level permanent staff at the Ministry of Public Health. Supawat and others would also explore the possibility of obtaining some sort of royal blessing for the hepatitis eradication program and for a local manufacturing plant as well.[80]

Task Force and PATH representatives began meeting with a variety of different groups whose support might help get the project off the ground. Mahoney met with the Communicable Disease Control Division staff of the Ministry of Public Health, among them Dr. Supamit, who had attended the earlier meeting with Wilde and Douglas. Supamit told Mahoney that the National Hepatitis B Advisory Committee had met that very morning and given Supamit the responsibility for coordinating a master plan for hepatitis B. The plan would be a position paper that laid out the options for the Ministry's consideration.

Mahoney was also told that the Ministry did not want a demonstration program that would be ended in a few years, since in the past such programs had raised expectations and left people angry and frustrated. Mahoney explained that the Task Force was in agreement on this point and suggested that they begin to call it a demonstration program rather than a "model" project, to emphasize that it was to lead to a wide-scale, national implementation of the program.

Mahoney also informed the Ministry staff that if the Task Force were to operate in Thailand, it would use the Ministry of Public Health as its first reference point, since they would have responsibility for implementation of the hepatitis B program. Still, the Task Force would also seek to work with other groups, including Mahidol and Chulalongkorn Universities and the Thai Red Cross.[81] Later, Mahoney met with Supamit's superior, Dr. Teera Ramasoota, Deputy Director of the Communicable Disease Control Division, the man most directly concerned with decisions regarding hepatitis B and the Expanded Programme for Immunization (EPI) in Thailand. Teera expressed support for Task Force efforts and felt that having a representative of the Task Force present at the next meeting of the National Hepatitis B Advisory Committee would be useful.[82]

Mahoney next met with President Natth of Mahidol University, who requested reassurance that the Task Force would not work exclusively with the Ministry of Public Health. Mahoney told Natth that one of the benefits of the Task Force's independence and its association with PATH was that it did not have to work only with the government. Natth said that it was possible that the Princess Chulakorn Foundation might contribute money to the hepatitis B vaccine demonstration program. He also let Mahoney know that the Princess was a scientist, and that he had been her mentor while she was at the University.[83]

Mahoney later saw the Dean and Vice Dean of Chulalongkorn University. It was clear that the University was anxious to be involved in any Task Force–sponsored project. These officials pointed out that the medical school had established field capabilities in both rural and urban areas and could assist the vaccine program in either locale. The Dean also said that the University had established its own Task Force on Hepatitis B in 1985; this group had met regularly since then, but had not yet come up with any specific recommendations on how to proceed.[84]

When Mahoney spoke with Drs. Chaivej and Supawat of the Red Cross, they expressed their hope that the Task Force would assist them in conducting a feasibility study for the transfer of Dutch vaccine technology to Thailand. (Earlier, PATH had conducted such a study on rabies vaccine for the Red Cross.) They then talked of the role the Red Cross could play in the demonstration project. The Red Cross representatives wanted to locate funds that would allow them to donate the vaccine as part of their movement toward establishing local production that could supply the future national immunization program.[85]

The Thai Government Agrees to Set Up a Model Hepatitis B Project

A month after these preparatory meetings were held with Mahoney, a second set of conferences involving the same groups was arranged for Task Force members James Maynard and Ian Gust. At the meeting with Dr. Teera of the Communicable Disease Control Division the two were invited to make a presentation to the National Hepatitis B Advisory Committee. The presentation resulted in a major breakthrough for the Task Force—the Committee decided unanimously to adopt a policy of mass hepatitis B immunization of all newborns by 1992. In the five years before that date, one of two strategies would be employed: if no external assistance was available the Ministry would use its money to screen pregnant women and immunize only newborns of carrier mothers; if external assistance (from the International Task Force) was provided for vaccine procurement, a phased program for immunizing all newborns would be begun.[86]

Teera also told Maynard that the Thai Red Cross's interest in local production would be an integral part of the national plan. Teera felt that Dr. Chaivej of the Red Cross, in particular, should be given credit for the National Committee's quick response, because although he was not a member of the committee, he had attended its last two sessions and announced his intention to produce hepatitis B vaccine at the National Blood Center. He then challenged the Committee to come up with a plan that would make the vaccine available at no cost to the users.[87]

At a later meeting, Dr. Chaivej told Maynard and Gust that the hepatitis B production feasibility study could begin at any time and stated that he had asked the Dutch Red Cross for a commitment to train Thai staff in the Netherlands. (Within a month the Dutch withdrew their offer.) Chaivej also expressed his desire to involve the Department of Medical Sciences of the Ministry of Public Health because this would create a personal link with that crucial regulatory body.[88]

Maynard and Gust also met with Drs. Natth and Charas of Mahidol and Chulalongkorn Universities. Both academics again expressed their desire to get involved with the Task Force and the hepatitis B project. Natth announced his intention to launch a hepatitis B immunization program in one of the southern provinces. He expressed his strong support for Task Force work and suggested that the model project be launched on the King's sixtieth birthday. He also proposed that the University do the work of the model program. Maynard and Gust responded that they would have to be guided by the Ministry of Public Health, but that there would be a role for the universities to play. (Ultimately, the universities played a very minor role in the project, which angered and alienated important and well-connected people, including President Natth at Mahidol. The problem was that the universities wanted to conduct studies in their scholarly areas of interest, while the Task Force felt it had passed the stage of basic research and needed to move on to the problems of practical implementation.)

At this point things were moving fast and well on the hepatitis vaccine front, though a number of outstanding issues had to be decided before the model program could be launched. First, a local coordinating committee from the Ministry, including a principal investigator, had to be selected. It already appeared that Dr. Supamit would be chosen, and that a group of Communicable Disease Control Division officials would participate in the protocol development work. Second, calculations of in-kind contributions (i.e., working space, staff, and salaries) from the Ministry of Public Health had to be made. Third, a memorandum of understanding between the Ministry and the Task Force had to be signed once the protocols were written and approved. Fourth, a serology laboratory, probably within the Department of Medical Sciences of the Ministry of Public Health, needed to be established.[89]

In addition, the role the two universities would play in the project had to be determined. The universities had a great desire to be included, and the Ministry had no objections to allowing them to participate. While they would play no role in vaccine delivery, they would possibly participate in small-scale research, operational research, training, support, and follow-up. Development of educational and training materials (a PATH specialty) might also involve the universities. Lastly, PATH had to provide assistance to the Thai Red Cross for its feasibility study of local vaccine production. The fight against hepatitis B in Thailand was finally going into high gear.

An Outside Catalyst for the Hepatitis B Model Program in Thailand

The Task Force now had two separate but closely interrelated projects in Thailand. The first was the construction and implementation of the model program as a preparatory step for a future national hepatitis B immunization effort, and the second was the provision of assistance to the Thai Red Cross in obtaining vaccine technology so that it could ultimately become the supplier for the public sector.

Setting up the Thai model program was the Task Force's most important goal and its most significant victory. It acted as the indispensable catalyst for the Thai bureaucracy, enabling it to function more effectively on this issue. The Thais had the skilled people, the facilities, and the ability to tackle the hepatitis problem successfully, but they needed an outside agency to help break the bureaucratic logjams and conflicts that had immobilized them.

As we have seen, the Thais had been actively working on the issue of hepatitis B for a number of years before the International Task Force existed. They had even set up a National Hepatitis B Committee to deal with the situation. The Committee members included the people most knowledgeable about the problem in Thailand. But the process of deliberation was slow and painstaking—and the Committee membership represented diverse and often conflicting viewpoints and interests. In its first year the Committee studied the situation. In the second year it recommended that hepatitis B be the first viral hepatitis to be controlled, with vaccination the major instrument for that control. The target population should be newborn and other risk groups. It recommended that the containment program should be implemented stepwise: first, by the screening of mothers and the immunization of the children of carriers, and second, by the gradual integration of the program into the regular EPI. In addition, the Committee recommended that the Ministry of Health support the goal of local production of vaccine.

These recommendations, however, were not made directly to the Minister but rather to the head of the Committee (i.e., the Director-General of the Communicable Disease Control Division), who screened all recommendations before they proceeded higher up the hierarchy. He was interested but suggested the problem be given more study, and a series of subcommittees were set up. All kinds of questions had to be investigated: How would it be possible to screen mothers in the countryside when the facilities were not in place? How could a sufficient number of test kits be obtained? Who would produce them? The subcommittees reported their deliberations, but the Director-General remained reluctant to set up the control program, citing its lack of economic feasibility. He would not pass the recommendations on to the Permanent Secretary (the highest civil servant in the Ministry), and thus they would not be presented to the Minister of Public Health (a political appointee).[90] A national program would have to be advocated by the Minister of Public Health.

The hepatitis B problem probably would have remained stalled at just this point for years without an outside push to move it forward. It was only with the appearance of the Task Force, and its funds waiting in the wings, that the Director-General decisively approved the recommendations.

The Protocol

The protocol for Thailand was in many ways like the proposal for Indonesia and thus was able to benefit from that earlier work.[91] The Task Force arranged for Dr. Violet How of Malaysia to help write the document, and Maynard was able to send his assistant, Mark Kane, as well. The protocol was written in the Thai Communicable Disease Control Division, and Kane took it with him to Atlanta for final polishing. It was then sent back to Thailand and presented to the Ministry. Later, the document was officially offered to the Task Force.

As in Indonesia, the Thai model program was designed to show that hepatitis B immunization could be successfully integrated into the EPI. In keeping with that goal, no program activity was to be carried out solely for the purpose of delivering hepatitis vaccine. The methods also had to be replicable in other regions of Thailand and in other developing countries. In addition, the program was structured to encourage the continuation of mass childhood vaccination at the end of the four-year project. The protocol also proposed to achieve an 85 percent success rate in delivering three doses of vaccine to infants in the target areas, to identify the major obstacles to administering vaccine (within seven days of birth) to infants born at home, and to achieve a 90 percent success rate in reporting births within seventy-two hours.[92]

The protocol called for the program to be managed by a team composed of representatives of the Thai Ministry of Public Health, the

International Task Force, and PATH. The Task Force would be represented by a Task Force liaison representative (Dr. Violet How) and PATH staff members from Bangkok and Seattle. A consultant from the U.S. CDC would also be part of the team.

The core program staff was to be led by the Principal Investigator, who would have responsibility for day-to-day operations, including personnel management, educational and training activities, data collection and analysis, and program evaluation. The Principal Investigator would be aided by a Co-Principal Investigator and technical assistants. Given Thai realities, the Principal Investigator had to be an honorary position held by the Director-General of the Communicable Disease Control Division, with the Co-Principal Investigator, Dr. Supamit, actually functioning as head of the program. PATH was to provide administrative and financial services for the project, and all funds for the program were to be channeled through the offices of PATH in Seattle and Bangkok.

The Thai National Team Leader

The success of the model program depended to a large extent on the abilities and commitment of the Co-Principal Investigator, Dr. Supamit Chunsuttiwat. Supamit was an exceptionally capable and dedicated young man, an excellent representative of the new generation of bright, well-trained young Thais—the so-called technocratic elite whose education has involved spending time abroad. Supamit received his training in epidemiology at the CDC in Atlanta. He had the opportunity to observe firsthand the hepatitis B survey done in American Samoa, and he produced a cost analysis of hepatitis B in Thailand, under Mark Kane's supervision, as part of his Atlanta CDC thesis.[93] When he joined the Thai Ministry of Public Health he was placed on the National Hepatitis Committee, where he was kept up-to-date on the government's attempts to set up an effective containment program.

Supamit also had occasion to interact with PATH. In 1985 he presented his cost analysis of hepatitis B at Chulalongkorn University. His thesis was that at $2.50 a shot, immunization without screening would be more cost effective than any alternative policy. Henry Wilde found the work interesting and asked if he could show it to the Indonesians. Wilde also informed Supamit that PATH was interested in doing a model program in Thailand.[94] A year later Supamit, representing the Ministry of Public Health, was part of the Thai Hepatitis Action Group that met with PATH to discuss what steps could be taken to speed up the process and get the Task Force involved. Subsequently the National

Hepatitis Committee gave him the responsibility for preparing the master plan of hepatitis B options for their consideration.

Under Supamit's supervision the model program proceeded relatively smoothly, efficiently, and honestly. Problems that arose were studied and rectified. The Task Force and PATH had to use far less budgetary control in Thailand than they had in Indonesia. The Thais were quite frugal and avoided waste—sometimes to an extreme in the opinion of PATH people.[95] According to Wilde,[96] the Ministry of Public Health generally ran a tight system of regional hospitals, clinics, and centers, with the Thai character being quite rigid, if not compulsive, about doing things properly. Supamit himself[97] did not intend to be overly inflexible about vaccine supplies, but once Provincial Controllers were informed that the vaccine was expensive, they adopted a very strict position, scrupulously checking the number of vaccine receipts against the amount supplied. There was virtually no corruption in the project, partly because it was seen as an EPI program, and everyone knew that no one could profit from it in the private marketplace, and more specifically because of the powerful local commitment to the program. Low-level corruption in projects is more likely to appear in connection with time-limited, foreign-donor projects, which are seen as benefiting outsiders rather than the local population and its leaders.[98]

The ability of Supamit and PATH to control the project, and the willingness of the workers to obey them, was best illustrated when several individuals requested that an exception be made in the designation of the population eligible for vaccination. The protocol made it clear that only newborn babies were to be immunized in the target areas, but the health care workers carrying out the project wanted to vaccinate their own older children. The request was refused, and the workers, with few exceptions, accepted that refusal. (This situation contrasts markedly with the situation in Jordan, where a planned model program for hepatitis B vaccination found doctors and nurses unwilling to cooperate because they did not receive the vaccine first.)[99] Supamit and Donald Douglas (of PATH) did not feel they had to buy off local workers to make the program successful.

Increasing Support from the Thai Government

Once the hepatitis program began it became clear that commitment existed not only at the local level but at the highest governmental levels as well. Initially, there had been no firm government guarantee of support for the program after the four-year demonstration project was ended. Thus, Supamit and his co-workers had only a limited time (provided by Task Force money) to prove that hepatitis B containment was worthwhile. The Task Force agreed to pay for the vaccine—which in the first year amounted to 90 percent of the program's expenses—and the program's administrative costs. But, unexpectedly, in the second year the Task Force did not pay for the vaccine, its official reason being that its donors had required that they discontinue this funding. The actual reason for the change in policy was that the Task Force felt its resources were limited, and that the need for the establishment of model programs in other parts of the world (especially Africa) had to take precedence over continuing subsidies to a more economically developed country. Task Force members believed that the Thais were committed enough and had sufficient resources to pick up the expense. This maneuver was a gamble, but the Task Force was willing to take the risk. Douglas, now the head of the local office, pleaded with the Task Force not to adopt such a tactic for fear that the project would collapse and all its work come to nothing.[100] His fear was not far from Supamit's anxiety that the loss of funds would trigger a significant cutback in the program.[101]

Instead, in the second year the Director-General decided to expand the program to two additional provinces—using the government's own money. The Task Force's gamble paid off. The increased support resulted from the fact that the actualization of the model project had radically changed the psychological perspective of top Thai bureaucrats. Despite all the years of governmental committee meetings dealing with hepatitis B, there had been a lack of political will at the highest levels to institute concrete action.[102] According to President Natth of Mahidol University, this was because a game of musical chairs existed among the top leadership in the Health Department, as people rotated into and out of office:

No one stayed long enough to know the situation. . . . I told every new [Permanent] Secretary and Director General that they would have a bad political situation if they ignored hepatitis B—everyone [in the countries] around [Thailand] was doing it. . . . [In addition] the National Health Plan was too rigid to adjust to the hepatitis B technological breakthroughs. They were overly focused on primary health care—and hepatitis B was seen as high tech— [which was] a mistake. Primary health care vs. high-tech is not all or nothing. Developing countries cannot ignore high-tech. Health is the most international thing. You can't just isolate yourself in primary health care. [There is no shame in it because] you actively react to Western Advisors, [you're] not just passive.[103]

The Task Force's initiative successfully changed the situation and pushed the government into a commitment to self-generated action.

Supamit had assumed that the Thai team would require a fair

amount of technical scientific assistance during the project from the Task Force advisor, Violet How, but he found this not to be the case. After the initial input from Dr. How, and additional pointers from Maynard, the Thais had few problems they could not handle by themselves. They were quite capable scientifically, but they needed more help on administrative matters—which they received from the local PATH office in Bangkok.[104]

The Local PATH Office and the Model Program

Donald Douglas, as head of the PATH office, saw his job as actualizing the Task Force's commitment on a daily basis and providing an administrative support system for the Thai team. Because of the great distances and expenses involved, the Task Force and PATH-Seattle were able to send emissaries only at infrequent intervals. Although Violet How lived close by in Malaysia, she was overworked and found it hard to spare time for the project.[105] The local office, however, was ready and willing to fill the gap. Douglas, while highly impressed with the Ministry of Public Health's commitment and abilities in carrying out the program, felt the success of the project nevertheless required the constant involvement of his office. PATH could supply the extra staff, time, and effort that the Ministry, with the best of intentions, simply did not have. The local people, whether the Principal Investigator or university or government personnel, had other responsibilities beyond just the model program. They often simply did not have the time that was required. If a vaccine shipment ended up at the wrong airport, or there was a question of whether vaccine had frozen while stored, PATH had the personnel to respond. A multitude of administrative questions and problems arose that required a comment, extra money, or a fast evaluation which PATH-Bangkok could provide. Douglas requested regular meetings with the Thai team to keep in touch and provide assistance. To Supamit, Douglas's administrative help was vital. He was also impressed by his understanding of and sensitivity to the Thai system.[106]

The local office maintained continuous and regular dialogues with government officials to bolster the sense of partnership between the Task Force and PATH and the Thais. It also worked to lay the groundwork for visits by Task Force and PATH-Seattle staff. Often, painstaking preparation was required to make possible the swift and smooth agreements that came out of those brief trips. Douglas felt he had to keep up with the changing political scene and the constantly changing cast of political characters—who was in and who was out in Thailand—in order to brief visitors such as Maynard and Mahoney. It was as important to know who was angry and insulted, or required a dinner invitation, as it was to know the substantive issues about the project. Attention to cultural and political sensitivity was vital, and the local office saw the provision of such information as one of its major jobs. It was especially important that the Thais feel that they were the owners of the model project (and have others perceive it this way as well). The Task Force and PATH had to be seen as helping, rather than dominating or leading, the Thais. Achieving all of this took a great amount of diplomacy and care.[107]

Both the Ministry of Public Health and the PATH office were determined to make sure that the model project worked, and was seen to work, for the benefit of the Thai population. They were very concerned about practical details and did not leave anything to chance. This was nowhere better illustrated than in the careful plans they made for launching the project. They chose to present the program as a gift on the sixtieth birthday of the King of Thailand. The sixtieth birthday, as the fifth cycle of twelve years, was considered to be especially auspicious by Buddhists. The ceremony would be jointly organized by the three concerned parties (PATH, the Ministry of Public Health, and the Thai Red Cross). However, as one memo noted regarding the opening proceedings,

No baby vaccination . . . will be demonstrated during the launch ceremony for fear of creating a false impression among the TV viewers that the national mass HB [hepatitis B] immunization is [about to] . . . start. People may flock to the Government health outlets asking for free vaccinations. . . . Another reason for no baby vaccination is that the newborn brought out of the hospital just for demonstration may contract pneumonia. If unfortunately that show baby dies of the disease a few days later, it will be a tragedy to everyone concerned and a . . . big issue for the press.[108]

The three groups wanted the press and the people on their side, running neither ahead of them nor behind them.

Limited Educational Aspects of the Otherwise Successful Model Hepatitis B Project

In the years after the model project was established, it proved itself a great success. Coverage was excellent. Hepatitis B vaccination was integrated into the EPI without hindering its effectiveness in any way. (EPI coverage was already so high that it was not possible to tell whether hepatitis B vaccination helped increase coverage, as it had in Indonesia.)[109] Most importantly, it convinced the government to go ahead with a national immunization program for the whole country, thus achieving the Task Force's primary goals.

In keeping with the commitment by the Task Force and PATH to perfecting the model projects, both to improve current performance and to aid future efforts, they set up a large-scale evaluation of the information, education, and communication (IEC) aspects of the Thai program in 1990. PATH established the research team, but it was headed by an academic from Mahidol University, in collaboration with other researchers from Chiang-mai University. The researchers were allowed total independence, and the leaders were given carte blanche to criticize.[110]

The situation the researchers found in Thailand was similar to that in Indonesia: the project was quite successful in delivering vaccine, but not as a result of the educational efforts. For Supamit and members of the Ministry of Public Health team, this was neither surprising nor unacceptable, but the Task Force and PATH were not happy with this situation and wanted to improve it.

The evaluation found a large number of problems in the education and communication efforts. In both provinces where the model project was administered there was no clear policy on the distribution of printed manuals, and they were not received by the target population. Because health personnel were often overwhelmed by the variety of Ministry of Public Health pamphlets available and confused as to which items went with which project, they often reacted with disillusionment and disinterest. Recorded instructional tapes dealing with hepatitis B were often not available in the villages, or if they were, there was no one to play them.

More important, when the researchers watched the general EPI being given, they found that "at most places . . . no explanations were made on the kinds of vaccine given, for which diseases, and why it was given."[111] Vaccine education seemed to get lost in the flood of information presented to mothers. Even when mothers asked for information they often were only handed printed material rather than a personal communication.

In Focus Group Discussions (FGDs) mothers were often unaware of hepatitis B or did not consider it a severe disease. Nevertheless, most of the women brought their infants to be immunized. The researchers were told by a vaccinator that "mothers may not associate the vaccine with the disease—they just believe that vaccines are good for the baby because the doctor said so."[112] Mothers' trust in health care workers was found to be a significant factor in many investigations, and there existed as well a widespread belief that "vaccination is a universal protection against diseases for children."[113]

Health care personnel gave priority to hepatitis B vaccination and did more follow-ups than before, but they did not recognize that mothers needed in-depth knowledge about the EPI diseases, nor that such knowledge could help increase coverage. The workers themselves often were fairly ignorant about hepatitis B: they did not read the manual themselves or felt insecure about the understanding they received from the brief training periods they had participated in.

On the plus side, the researchers found that provincial health personnel did give the program high priority, and that they emphasized its importance at every monthly meeting with the chiefs of the district health centers and directors of the district hospitals. The provincial health officers sensed the importance of the project because it was closely monitored by project administrators from the central Communicable Disease Control Division office. This attitude was very helpful for the program.

The results of the independent study came as something of a shock to the Task Force and PATH. The tone of the study was very downbeat. There was a feeling that the researchers had been overly critical, but that nevertheless major problems did exist which had to be addressed.[114] Fortunately, these problems could be resolved. As a result of the evaluation, PATH decided to alter the structure of training and the types of educational materials used. Much greater emphasis was placed on staff training and the education of health personnel. In addition, the old system of having provincial staff train district staff and district staff train subdistrict staff was replaced by a system wherein all personnel in the province trained together. Group discussions with a problem-solving approach were recommended to take the place of lectures.

The printed material was reevaluated as well. PATH had prepared very costly books that were both physically heavy and very expensive looking. In the eyes of the Thai distributor, the books were too good to give to mothers! As a result of the evaluation, PATH revamped the whole print campaign. Less costly materials were used so that no one would feel he was giving something valuable away. The book was in fact condensed into a brochure, and more nonwritten media aids were utilized. PATH personnel sat down with the Ministry and decided exactly what people needed to know. The earlier effort had emphasized "What is Hepatitis B"; the new emphasis was not on "what is it," but on the more practical *when* to go and get the shots. Since the mothers already supported vaccination, they did not need to be educated on technical issues. From Douglas's standpoint the consultant's report was very useful and demonstrated the vital importance of an independent assessor, even if at first he was rather embarrassed by its findings, PATH was able to maintain its commitment to IEC work and to benefit from its mistakes.[115] The evaluation, however, made clear that the IEC materials, even at their best, could never replace personal interactions between health staff and mothers, but only supplement it.[116]

For the Task Force and PATH members the fact that "the level of knowledge among mothers about the diseases and regular course of EPI vaccinations is considerably lower than one would expect given the high coverage rates of the Thai EPI program"[117] was very unsettling, just as it had been in Indonesia. The Task Force and PATH were pragmatic enough to use the customary acceptance of authority in Southeast Asia to achieve their project goals, but they neither believed nor wanted to believe that long-term success could be built upon such a basis. Education was still seen as being of fundamental importance.

Supamit and his team, however, were far less concerned with the educational problems than the Task Force was:

About mother-education, we weren't [initially] clear what they thought about the EPI—so we welcomed the idea of the IEC aspect [of the project]. . . . After the second year assessment it became clear that the mothers were not knowledgeable [about EPI/hepatitis B] but [rather they were simply] trusting. We were happy. Maynard was not happy. He felt for sustainability they must know [about hepatitis B]. We were happy with that [approach] too—because we wanted 100% [vaccine coverage, rather than the 90% we could get without an elaborate educational effort, but] . . . the last 10% would be very difficult [and could benefit from it]. The Thais, thus, were not converted to Maynard's view of education.[118]

The Thai social structure worked on the basis of hierarchy and respect for authority. For many Thais the system worked and did not require the mass educational efforts that the Task Force and PATH saw as vital. Such efforts clearly were not indispensable here.

The Task Force felt that education of village health workers, as opposed to mothers, was crucial, based on the assumption that in Thailand, as in Indonesia, most births took place at home. In reality, the vast majority of births (90 percent)[119] took place in hospitals, which greatly simplified the process of vaccination. The Task Force only realized this fact as the project progressed, though Supamit reported that he and his team were aware of this from the beginning, and it was one of the reasons they were not concerned about education.[120]

The Choice of Vaccine for the Model Project and the Task Force's Relationship to Cheil

One other source of trouble in the Thai model program revolved around the vaccine to be used—which was initially the Cheil vaccine. The original determination of which company would supply the vaccine to the project (and possibly later transfer its technology as well) put Task Force members in an awkward position. The Ministry of Public Health and the Thai Red Cross asked them to review the various options available and make a recommendation. In response they produced a report[121] that reviewed the pluses and minuses of each of the nine hepatitis B vaccine manufacturers and argued that Cheil best met Thailand's requirements. The reasoning was quite straightforward: Cheil offered the best price, and its production process required the smallest capital investment, since it did not use a large amount of expensive hardware and was technically the simplest process to reproduce.

The problem was that while the report was persuasive on the surface, many Thai observers assumed that Cheil's preeminence had been a foregone conclusion. In Thailand, PATH had been perceived for years as an agent of Cheil, and the Task Force was seen as the heir to that relationship.

Indeed, among the Thais, as among the Indonesians, the Task Force was not seen as an entirely independent entity at all, but more a creation and creature of PATH, an organization with which they were familiar by virtue of its long-term presence in Southeast Asia. Ian Gust might worry about who was the tail and who was the dog between the two organizations, but the Thais tended to feel that the reality was obvious. The Task Force, with leaders such as Maynard and Prince, enjoyed a prestige to which PATH could not lay claim; the real power was seen to issue from the subordinate organization. Any claim that the Task Force, unlike PATH, was not intimately tied to Cheil would have been seen as ludicrous given the relationship Alfred Prince and the NYBC shared with that company.

Thus the Task Force's vaccine recommendation was seen as tainted, and assumed to be financially self-serving. Unfortunately, PATH and the Task Force could do little to counteract these perceptions in Thailand, any more than they could do so in Indonesia. The Task Force, as we have seen, had been created because of the existence of the Cheil vaccine, and the methodology Prince had developed for it was a key to its applicability in developing countries. Those who have the benefit of unrestricted access to PATH and Task Force records can see that both groups objectively considered all manufacturers as potential sources of technology. The Task Force and PATH finally chose Cheil based upon the merits of the case, uninfluenced by any financial benefit to themselves. For those without access to organizational files, however, there was no way to eliminate the underlying suspicion about the Task Force's motivation. The view of Dr. Prayura Kunasol, Deputy Director of the Thai Communicable Disease Control Division in 1992, is probably representative:

In my heart I have some doubt about Cheil. But I could not argue against it on scientific grounds. . . . I could not argue . . . because of cost. . . . I had to accept it. I had to accept it for the sake of the kids. [But] I suspected Cheil and PATH. I did not have evidence to argue openly. [Of course] it is a normal event that when you ask individuals involved, you will get a distorted view because of their involvement.[122]

Not having the evidence to argue openly did not prevent people from making those views known in a less direct fashion—especially within the Thai bureaucracy, where indirection is a way of life.

The Thais accepted the Task Force's recommendation, but not without severe reservations. Those reservations were heightened by their distrust of any Korean company that acted as a source of a high-technology product. The fact that the Korean vaccines were not sold in the United States caused concern among the Thais. Indeed, the fact that recombinant DNA (rather than plasma) vaccines were used in the United States was constantly raised as an objection to Task Force support for the use of plasma-derived vaccines in Asia.[123] The Task Force feasibility report tried to take note of this attitude by saying that "the vaccine production process used by Cheil was actually developed by the New York Blood Center (NYBC) and the CLB [Dutch Red Cross]."[124] The report emphasized that Cheil produced the vaccine under license from the NYBC and was subject to supervision by it. Unfortunately, this gave the impression that the Task Force had greater influence over Cheil than it actually possessed.[125]

The reality was that Prince and Maynard could exhort, threaten, plead with, or entice Cheil, but they could not control it. The men running Cheil were superior businessmen in the sugar industry, but were fairly inept at selling pharmaceuticals. When questions about the efficacy of the vaccine arose, they were slow to deal with them or to offer proof of the quality of their product. This was especially harmful when widespread doubts about the acceptability of the Cheil vaccine arose in the period after the inauguration of the Thai model program.

Thai fears about the quality of Cheil vaccine occurred both at the provincial level (where some health workers refused to use it) and at higher governmental levels. Donald Douglas[126] felt that while the core Ministry of Public Health team steadfastly maintained its support of Cheil, lower-level staff and the Thai academic community were increasingly hostile. Those Thais who were still sympathetic to Cheil strongly urged that Prince come to Thailand and speak to the National Hepatitis Committee to put their minds at ease. The situation was quickly becoming critical.

To make matters worse, Dr. Praphan of the Thai Red Cross completed a study[127] comparing the Cheil vaccine with the Merck, Pasteur, and Dutch vaccines, and concluded that the Cheil vaccine was simply inadequate. His findings were especially damaging to the Task Force's position, and the fact that Praphan's methodology and interpretation were flawed was not in itself enough to nullify the harm the report inflicted. The Task Force felt it was vital that Cheil make a special effort to bolster its scientific claims by immediately releasing data supportive of its vaccine's efficacy and by initiating new studies of the vaccine. But Cheil was slow in reacting to protect the scientific reputation of its vaccine,[128] just as it was remiss in responding to constant reminders from PATH that it must register its product in Thailand and find a local partner if it had a genuine desire to establish itself as an ongoing business there.[129]

Cheil's uncooperativeness ultimately reached the point where the Task Force was compelled to ask the company whether it had any real commitment to selling hepatitis B vaccine outside Korea, since "there have been times in which we believe we have seen indications that Cheil is less than fully committed to the international market."[130]

The problem with Cheil, at least as far as Donald Douglas could see, was that the idealism that had played such a pivotal role in committing Cheil to $1 a dose for hepatitis B vaccine in the first place had come primarily from Shin Seung-il of Eugene Tech, who was more a visionary than an entrepreneur. It was he who had obtained the vital patronage and support of Samsung's chairman, B. C. Lee. When Lee died, Shin lost his leverage, and Cheil management narrowed its focus to short-range questions of immediate profit and loss.[131]

A major crisis arose a number of months after the Thai model project had become operational, when Cheil temporarily ran out of hepatitis B vaccine. Its response to an urgent request to push up its production schedule was negative. The Task Force was forced to turn around quickly and recommend that the Thais switch from Cheil to Korean Green Cross Corporation (KGCC) vaccine, which the Thais did.

The switch from Cheil to KGCC vaccines in the model project offered the possibility that the Task Force and PATH would finally rid themselves of the nagging suspicions that their relationship with Cheil was in some way a self-serving one. (A similar opportunity arose in Indonesia when the KGCC won the original international bid and tender.) Unfortunately, this valuable opportunity was lost due to a clerical misstep.

Over the course of KGCC's negotiations for the right to transfer hepatitis B vaccine technology to Thailand, KGCC representatives included in their letter to PATH a postscript offering to donate 20 percent of any royalties they received to PATH, if they obtained the contract. Mahoney responded to the offer by requesting that KGCC instead donate the money to the Thai Red Cross or to the government; PATH itself could not accept it. When duplicates of the documents were sent to the Red Cross, the letter containing the postscript was included, but the letter refusing the offer was not. To the Thais it appeared the Task Force's recommendation had simply been bought by another Korean company. When Maynard heard about the error, he tried to undo the damage by explaining the situation, but this did not satisfy or convince the Thais. They did, however, politely act as if they accepted his explanation.[132]

Attempts to Transfer Hepatitis B Production Technology to Thailand

The first goal of the Task Force was to create a successful Thai hepatitis B model project that would ultimately lead to a nationwide immunization program; its second aim was to help in the transfer of vaccine-manufacturing technology to Thailand. This latter goal was consistent with PATH's long-standing interest in fostering local production, which had motivated its original contacts with Alfred Prince and the Cheil Sugar Company and energized its original efforts to create the Task Force.

As we have seen, Prince and Maynard were also personally committed to the idea of local vaccine production in Third World countries. They both believed that the continued monopoly of high technology in the West (and Japan) was inherently wrong and dangerous, that it was fed by lingering racism which it in turn perpetuated. The idea that developing countries could not produce quality vaccines, Maynard argued, tended to become a self-fulfilling prophecy insofar as new (Asian) companies were forced to meet unnecessarily strict vaccine standards set by WHO. True independence and national pride demanded that developing countries be able to produce their own vaccines.[133] (Mahoney for a long time was also personally supportive of the goal of technology transfer to developing countries, but his commitment was based primarily on straight economic cost-benefit criteria. The different philosophical bases underlying the three men's positions ultimately led to significant discord among them.)

The conflict between those committed to promoting Third World independence in vaccine manufacturing and those hostile to such a venture was well illustrated in the rival interpretations of the Task Force's activities in the developing world that appeared in two prestigious periodicals—one published in Europe (*Nature*) and the other in Asia (*Far East Review*).

The *Nature* article,[134] pointedly titled "Hepatitis B Vaccine Contract

Goes to Untested Product," was little more than a bullet aimed at the heart of the Task Force and at the ambitions of the developing nations it championed. The author informed the reader that SmithKline and Merck, both makers of high-technology recombinant DNA vaccines, had lost a major international supply contract to a small Korean pharmaceutical company, KGCC, a situation that was the brain child of the International Task Force on Hepatitis B Immunization. While China, Taiwan, and South Korea did indeed produce plasma-derived vaccines,

[n]one of these vaccines has been tested for safety and efficacy by an independent regulatory authority. Health professionals now worry that in their zeal to get the vaccines to countries that need it . . . the task force may be endorsing a potentially substandard product. . . . The task force . . . took the unorthodox step of declaring all vaccines acceptable if approved by the national regulatory authority of the countries of origin. . . . Such is the demand for a cheap vaccine in many parts of South-East Asia that some countries are willing to take a gamble rather than wait for the major companies to lower their price.[135]

The fact that this article appeared in the prestigious journal *Nature* gave its indictment wide circulation and great credibility. The implication was clear: local Asian production risked the lives of the population, whereas Western products did not. Task Force leaders immediately challenged the facts of the article and protested *Nature*'s willingness to publish such misleading and misinformed analysis under its influential auspices.

A clear reply to this attack came two years later when the *Far East Review*[136] published a story on the same topic but under a radically different heading: "The Price Is Right: Cheap Hepatitis Vaccine Offers Immunization Breakthrough." It presented a markedly positive image of the production of hepatitis B vaccine in China and Korea and of the Task Force's price-shattering achievement in Indonesia. For Maynard the two clashing articles captured the essence of the fight between the East and the West over the maintenance of Euro-American technological supremacy, with the *Far East Review* clearly rejecting Western arrogance. Maynard relished the clear confrontation that was so startlingly presented by the two journals.[137]

The Thai Red Cross as a Partner in Transferring Vaccine Processing and Production Technology

As far as the Task Force could see, of all the groups interested in the transfer of hepatitis B technology, the Thai Red Cross appeared the most likely to carry it off successfully. When the Dutch Red Cross withdrew its offer to transfer technology to the organization in 1987, the Task Force was asked to step in and help find an alternative source.

It proceeded, not unexpectedly, to suggest Cheil, as both vaccine provider to the Thai model project and source for the technology transfer. Over the next two years the Task Force and PATH put extensive effort into analyzing how best the second undertaking could be arranged.

One difficulty they faced was that the Red Cross Society was divided into different divisions, and the two parts most concerned with vaccine technology were often pitted against each other as rivals. The Task Force's main contacts were with the Red Cross Institute, with which Henry Wilde was closely associated. Drs. Supawat and Praphan were the key figures in that group. The Institute was concerned with the processing of vaccine, not its actual production. In the first stage of technology transfer, vaccine produced abroad would be imported in bulk and then repacked into smaller vials. This repackaging would require the construction of a sterile filling facility, which would necessitate careful planning regarding building design, air-handling requirements, the recruitment of skilled personnel, and the appropriation of relevant equipment. Maintenance of sterile conditions and adequate quality control would require the establishment of a sophisticated, high-technology plant and operation.[138] The problem the Red Cross Institute faced was that, like most government organizations, it paid very low salaries. The most skilled people could not be attracted or kept for long periods with such pay. Those who did stay had to have second jobs to make ends meet. To attract the skilled workers the project needed the Red Cross would have to find some way to modify its pay schedule, or the venture would fail.[139] (This problem existed for both processing and production of vaccine.)

Not only did the Red Cross have to pay salaries competitive with the private sector, they also needed a private company as a partner to obtain large-scale private sector distribution of their product. The Task Force feasibility study showed that without private sector sales the project would not be economically workable.[140] The key benefit of private sector sales was that profits from it could be used to help subsidize the public sector. This was in fact the mechanism that private pharmaceutical companies used to supply the United Nations Children's Fund (UNICEF) with the inexpensive EPI vaccines.[141]

The Task Force view of the fundamental importance of salaries and private sector involvement was neither new nor unique to it, but rather consistent with the view expressed years earlier by Dr. Praphan, Science Director of the Red Cross, in discussions he had with PATH representative Henry Wilde. Wilde recounted:

When I asked . . . whether he thought that the decision makers at the Thai Red Cross would want to do this [technological transfer of hepatitis vaccine production] as an internal project of the Thai Red Cross, he said that this would be impossible. . . . [F]irst of all financing would not be available, the business know-how is not there and, above all, the workers would not be of sufficient calibre to be able to guarantee success due to low government salaries. He said that this type of venture would have to be a private one, though the Thai Red Cross would want to have a portion of the action. . . . [There would have to be] a private company located in the Thai Red Cross compound, perhaps on a lease basis, and operating the plan with the . . . Red Cross providing technical support, the blood, and scientific consultants.[142]

But as it developed, the Red Cross did not ultimately take this position. It was willing neither to raise salaries nor have a private sector partner.

As the Task Force came close to arranging substantive talks between the Institute and Cheil, Dr. Supawat suggested that some of the basic assumptions of the feasibility study be radically changed. First, he wanted the recommendation for a private partner removed; the Red Cross could sell the vaccine itself. Second, he felt that to the extent that private market sales materialized, the Red Cross and not the Ministry of Public Health should benefit from the cost savings that were generated; there should be no automatic subsidy to the Ministry. In addition, the Red Cross wanted to reduce the training costs charged by Cheil, since far less training was required for packaging workers than for production personnel. (Actual hepatitis B vaccine production would be under the control of the Red Cross's National Blood Center, the Institute's rival, and the Institute wanted nothing to do with the Center's work.)[143] In fact, the Red Cross leadership did not feel any need for Cheil to supervise their packaging of the bulk vaccine.[144]

The Task Force and PATH were appalled. They did not believe the venture could possibly succeed under such conditions. They feared that without private sector sales (and the royalties they generated) Cheil would lose interest or demand a very big up-front transfer fee. Without the profits it produced, and the resulting subsidy to the Ministry, the government would not be able to afford a mass immunization program. In addition, without the intimate involvement of Cheil staff in training and supervision, the level of quality control would be unacceptable, especially with the low-paid workers the Red Cross Institute envisioned. Even worse, the Red Cross was proposing to play politics with the Ministry of Public Health over the subsidy, and for the Task Force and PATH to side with such a tactic would be fatal to their relationship with the government.[145]

Since in preparing the feasibility study, the Task Force and PATH were simply acting as agents for the Thais, they felt they had to comply with the Red Cross Institute's demand for changes in the document, though they continued to press for what they saw to be more viable positions. Nevertheless, both PATH and the Task Force were primarily interested in

assist[ing] in making affordable hepatitis B vaccine available to developing countries . . . [and] only secondarily [were they] . . . interested in assisting in enhancing the vaccine handling capabilities of the Thai Red Cross . . . [since] the modifications made by Supawat . . . redirect the study much more to the second objective than the first.[146]

They could not assist a project in which the private sector sales were used entirely to the benefit of the manufacturer (i.e., the Red Cross) rather than the public. They would not support anything short of full disclosure to the Ministry, since it needed accurate information to determine what price to pay for the vaccine.[147]

Within a few months of these exchanges the Task Force presented the Thai Red Cross with its formal recommendations for technology transfer of hepatitis B vaccine production.[148] The report dealt with the two separate proposals the Red Cross had received—one from Cheil and one from the KGCC. The preferred company was still, despite all its problems, Cheil, but KGCC was seen as a close second. Cheil had a simpler and less expensive production process, which meant a lower capital investment and a more easily managed methodology. However, its lower cost was counterbalanced by its demand for a higher up-front payment. In other respects the Cheil offer was also inferior to that of KGCC. The Task Force thus suggested that the Red Cross make a series of counterproposals, essentially asking Cheil to meet the terms KGCC was offering. If Cheil did not agree, the Thais would switch companies, though only after it was agreed that KGCC would ultimately acquire the NYBC methodology and upgrade its relatively inefficient manufacturing process. The KGCC bid was seen as both a legitimate offer and a major bargaining tool to be used in negotiating with Cheil. The Task Force also recommended that the Red Cross not act alone in dealing with Cheil, but that it consult with the Ministry of Public Health.

The advisory report again strongly emphasized the fundamental importance of selling a portion of the production to the private sector; the proceeds would go to the Red Cross, which would thus be able to offer the Ministry a discount. KGCC (unlike Cheil) already had a private sector distributor in Thailand, and the report recommended that the Thais investigate this company to decide whether they would be comfortable working with it. KGCC wanted a royalty on all sales of vaccine—public and private—but the Task Force felt this would be incompatible with the goal of achieving the lowest possible vaccine price. The Task Force believed, however, that the company would be amenable to taking royalties only on private sector sales. In general the report suggested that the Red Cross exploit the situation created by having two rival bidders in order to get the best possible offer, though its preference was that Cheil end up the winner.[149]

At this point, Thai suspicions notwithstanding, the Task Force very clearly put local production (and the interests of the host country) above that of the Cheil Sugar Company. It not only advised the Red Cross to exert maximum pressure on Cheil, it also provided pressure of its own. Though the Task Force and PATH claimed to be simply "serving as friendly intermediaries"[150] between the two groups, their main loyalty was to the Thais—provided they did not subvert the larger goal of providing a cheap vaccine for mass immunization. They were aware, however, that both groups—Cheil and the Red Cross—were talking about undertaking a project with which neither had any extensive experience or expertise. Even Cheil had only been on the receiving end of technology transfer, not on the providing side. The Task Force realized that one or the other of the parties might get cold feet when they thought more deeply about the matter, though it was hoped this would not occur.[151]

Unfortunately, an epidemic of cold feet or at least second thoughts hit the participants within a very short time. Cheil was first to show it had lost interest in the enterprise. Mahoney described the situation quite succinctly:

It is clear that the previous public sector interest of Cheil has diminished if not disappeared all together. If Cheil were to be selected as the collaborator for production, Cheil would approach the project from almost totally a commercial point of view. . . . Cheil seems to have reduced its overall priority for hepatitis B vaccine. The company now sells some 14 vaccines and a large number of pharmaceutical products. . . . Thus Cheil is devoting its financial and intellectual energies to those products that have the greatest promise of rapid market growth.[152]

But KGCC's attitude was just the opposite of Cheil's. The president of that company, Mr. Huh Young-sup, was

sincerely committed to assisting the developing world to deal with hepatitis B control. He has a personal commitment that will stand as an insurance policy against project failure. We can expect him to do what is necessary to get things on track if major problems arise.[153]

Unfortunately, the National Blood Center, the division of the Red Cross charged with actually producing vaccine, was not interested in KGCC any more than in Cheil. The Thais increasingly seemed to want to go it alone. They felt that any technology transfer would be too expensive. According to one observer, "They [seem to] think they can simply rig-up some machinery on their own, get some donated Japanese equipment, read a few books, hire a couple of consultants and produce a vaccine."[154] When they were told by Donald Douglas that neither PATH nor the NYBC would assist a plan that lacked a core production technology, the Thais offered no compromise in response.[155] The claim by knowledgeable people in Thailand that the National Blood Center would not be able to hire staff with adequate capabilities to produce vaccine was seeming more and more credible.[156] Mahoney reached the point that he felt the idea of Red Cross vaccine production (as opposed to processing of imported vaccine) should be shelved. Instead, he believed they should move aggressively to get the Red Cross Institute to set up a sterile filling operation in collaboration with KGCC and that they then should explore the possibility of setting up a joint venture between the Red Cross and some private Thai firm to produce vaccine. PATH would be able to help find the money to develop the project, but Mahoney would not act until senior Red Cross management showed a strong commitment to such an effort, which so far they had not done.

There was a real danger that if the National Blood Center remained determined to produce vaccine on its own, there would be a disaster. As a result, not only would the Thais suffer, but the Task Force's international reputation and credibility would suffer as well. Some way to stop the National Blood Center from reinventing the wheel had to be found. Some thought that perhaps providing the money for KGCC's technical transfer fee would do the job.[157]

Unfortunately, according to Supawat of the Red Cross Institute, it was not economics that led the National Blood Center to attempt production without help, it was pride. They had the money but did not want Korean assistance. The Task Force's offer to pay the transfer costs would not be accepted for that reason. While an offer could be made to the top echelon of the Red Cross Society, the decision would still be left to the National Blood Center.[158]

The Red Cross Institute's interest in processing bulk vaccine looked much more promising. Indeed, the increasing probability of the failure of local production made the sterile vialing of bulk imported vaccine that much more attractive. It came as a surprise that, instead, the repackaging scheme also seemed to founder.[159]

Institutional Rivalries Block Transfer of Hepatitis B Vaccine Technology

In the end, the transfer of hepatitis B technology, whether via vaccine production or bulk processing, did not occur. The question is why.

There are a variety of explanations that shed light on the situation in Thailand and other developing countries, and highlight the problems faced by the Task Force in working in such complex environments.

The main reason PATH and the Task Force failed to help the Thais successfully produce hepatitis B vaccine was that they chose the wrong institutional vehicle—the Thai Red Cross—though they had no way of knowing their mistake. In fact, the choice of the Red Cross seemed a very astute and politically savvy one, providing proof of PATH's political and cultural sensitivity and expertise.

The Red Cross was a very important force in Thailand—it had royal patronage and intimate links to Chulalongkorn University, which was itself a major source of influence. The Red Cross possessed a variety of unique privileges, including the right to import unlicensed products that lacked Thai Food and Drug Administration approval. It was in some ways a small kingdom unto itself. The leaders of the Red Cross Institute and National Blood Center were intelligent and skilled professionals, men of the highest caliber whose ability and knowledge were equal to those of their peers anywhere in the world.

PATH, and later the Task Force, also had the good fortune of having Henry Wilde as a guide to Red Cross policies and politics. When he retired from the U.S. Foreign Service he became the first Westerner to be made a professor at a Thai university since the early twentieth century. He also had worked on rabies at the Red Cross Institute, an issue on which he was an international authority. One could not have asked for a better situation.

One Thai observer contends that by choosing the Red Cross, PATH had doomed its efforts because of the influence of Henry Wilde, who misled them into thinking he understood Thai power relationships better than he did.[160] But this charge is not convincing. When PATH came on the scene the Red Cross had already negotiated a hepatitis B vaccine agreement with the Dutch and was clearly the major player on this issue in Thailand, regardless of what Wilde or anyone else thought. The Red Cross's prior involvement basically dictated PATH policy, as it did for Thai government policy: the GPO, the Red Cross's logical competitor in vaccine production, bowed out of the competition in deference to the Red Cross's control of the playing field.[161]

The problem was that the Red Cross, while an important and prestigious organization, was simply not powerful enough within the Thai polity to accomplish the goal that PATH and the Task Force wished it to achieve. On the surface the chief weakness of the Thai Red Cross was its aversion to risk, but that attitude merely hid its more basic political weakness. The organization had all kinds of plans about hepatitis B, but it refused to undertake them without a government guarantee. In order for it to invest money in technology transfer, the Red Cross wanted to know that the government would buy the vaccine it produced in quantity, at a price that would protect the institution from losing money. It held to that demand consistently throughout the entire period of discussions and negotiations.

An early discussion between Wilde and Praphan casts a great deal of light on the Red Cross's ultimate failure. In discussing obstacles to be overcome for the project Praphan

immediately brought up the question that one would have [to] obtain a guarantee from the Thai Government that they would purchase the vaccine. . . . *He was probing me* to see whether I had any thoughts on this, and whether I thought it would be very likely that such advance assurance could be obtained from the Ministry of Health.[162]

Wilde's response was that from his experience and his questioning of government officials he did not think such an assurance could be obtained. The project would be initially a fairly risky investment, and at most the government would give the venture moral support.[163]

What is interesting in this exchange is not only the centrality of the demand for a guarantee, but the fact that Praphan, Scientific Director of the Red Cross, needed to probe Wilde to find out what the government's likely position would be. This situation was to be repeated more than once: ranking members of the Red Cross attempted to find out what was happening in their government by asking PATH people, or they requested that PATH lobby for the Red Cross when it met with the government. Such requests were a demonstration of significant political weakness.

The position taken by the government was that a guarantee was out of the question. Prayura, Deputy Director of the Communicable Disease Control Division, put it this way:

The Red Cross wanted to be sure that they could get back the money they invested in a fixed number of years. A guarantee they wanted. They are like a NGO [non-governmental organization]. They want a price and buyer; a fixed price. Those types of people were ignorant of the political situation. How can anyone say what government, with the same policy and budget will be there. No way! How can a civil servant make such a commitment for three, four, five years.[164]

Prayura's claim that no government would give long-term guarantees is less persuasive than the fact that no government would give such guarantees to an organization with the political weaknesses of the Red Cross. What the Red Cross received from the government was what foreigners often got: a series of polite responses that left them unaware (for years!) of the actual situation. According to President Natth of Mahidol University, the Red Cross got a classic "run-around for five years."[165] In the absence of the proper government connections, the Red Cross's only alternative was to take the risk on its own, but the organization did not have the necessary risk-taking spirit.

While the Red Cross's relative lack of political power clearly worked against it, it is also possible that other significant factors were at work. The GPO had politely refused to compete with the Red Cross over hepatitis B vaccine production as long as negotiations were active. However, once the Red Cross backed out the GPO felt free to enter the arena. The government position, as represented by Prayura, was that this was all quite straightforward:

Thai culture respects seniority and friendship. The venture was started by the Red Cross. It was not good for GPO to come in. Why compete? But if the Red Cross quit, then someone else might come. But this takes time. The current Director of the GPO was Deputy Director of the CDC [Communicable Disease Control Division] at the time the Red Cross was interested in local production. He waited until they left the field.[166]

Supamit, too, whose sincerity was very persuasive (but who was a subordinate of Prayura), contended that competition between the GPO and the Red Cross was not a factor—that, indeed, the Director of the GPO was very reluctant to get involved and wished the Red Cross well.[167]

This argument is presented not only by government officials but by outside observers as well. President Natth of Mahidol University contended that the GPO was the logical organization to produce vaccine all along, and that PATH's choice of the Red Cross had been an error from start to finish which simply, and unnecessarily, delayed the process of local production for years. The GPO would have been a better choice because it could act as a commercial firm and possessed the right to set up a semiprivate company or joint effort with a large pharmaceutical organization.[168] This arrangement would have provided the necessary know-how and supervision, as well as the higher salaries required to attract the most talented people.

Much of Natth's argument is clearly true: the GPO clearly could have side-stepped many of the Red Cross's handicaps, which the Task Force and PATH fruitlessly attempted to help them overcome. However, another difference existed between the two organizations that neither Natth nor Prayura mentioned. The Red Cross was a non-profit group, and to the extent that profits could be generated, they either would be passed on to the Ministry of Public Health in the form of a discount on the price of vaccine or kept in the Red Cross to benefit itself. The GPO, however, when it set up semiprivate firms, operated on a very different basis. If there were to be a profit much of it would be distributed to the staff and administrators of the GPO as individual bonuses. Vaccine production by the Red Cross personally benefited no one, while production by the GPO was a lucrative enterprise.[169] The arrangement created a rather strong incentive for the GPO to manufacture vaccine itself. In addition, the relations between the GPO and the Ministry of Public Health were close and harmonious, while those with the Red Cross tended to be rivalrous. Given this situation it is hard to believe that questions of financial gain by the bureaucracy had no effect on the final outcome.

Whatever the cause—GPO rivalry or the government's inability to give the type of long-term guarantee that the Red Cross demanded—the project died. The chief participants lost interest.

According to Wilde the project was already moribund when a final and unexpected blow came from the government. A letter was sent to the Red Cross saying that the government would not support the manufacture of any plasma-derived vaccine because of increasing doubts regarding its safety.[170] (Some Task Force members speculated that one of the big pharmaceutical companies had finally gotten to the government. This may be true, but the issue had already been decided before the letter was sent.)[171]

Disagreement Within the Task Force about the Desirability of Aiding Public Sector Manufacturing Ventures

The technology transfer failure in Thailand was a great disappointment for Task Force members Prince[172] and Maynard. Although the success of the model project and the government decision to start a national immunization program had been their main objectives, technology transfer had been a vital, even if secondary, goal.

Their feelings of frustration and defeat, however, were not shared by all in the Task Force. The issue of Thai production had brought to the surface an increasing division of opinion among the membership over local production of vaccine in the developing world. Ian Gust, always outspoken, wondered whether it made sense for the Task Force to continue its involvement with the issue since the group had already accomplished its goal of reducing the cost of the vaccine, and by the time the plasma-derived vaccine facilities were functioning, recombinant DNA or combined diphtheria-pertussis-tetanus-hepatitis B virus vaccines would have made plasma-derived vaccine obsolete. He also had doubts that the local facilities could ever produce a quality vaccine, and he questioned why the Task Force would want to risk its reputation in such increasingly risky ventures.[173]

Gust's doubts were strongly shared by Richard Mahoney. Mahoney also felt that the public sector in general could not successfully match the private sector in producing high-quality health products and services. Mahoney's disillusionment with the public sector (an opinion not shared by Gust) was potentially even more disruptive to smooth Task Force functioning than were qualms about technology transfer.

Mahoney's increasingly vocal hostility to hepatitis B vaccine local production marked a major change in attitude. Mahoney had been the one who had acted as the catalyst for the formation of the Task Force specifically because of his and PATH's interest in transferring hepatitis B vaccine technology to developing countries. Indeed, in the early period he had seen no legitimate obstacles to dissuade him from the desirability of that goal. His faith in its practicality had placed him at odds with many figures in the international health field who claimed it could not be done adequately. But as he became more involved in the process, he became increasingly skeptical about its feasibility and its necessity.

Part of Mahoney's change in attitude resulted simply from the fact that when the Task Force broke the price of the vaccine it had inadvertently made local production far less economically attractive. The increasingly lively competition in Asia among the biggest Euro-American pharmaceutical companies created a very favorable buyers' market for the vaccine, and it was not only Pasteur and SmithKline who entered the competition but even the previously aloof Merck. All of the companies were interested in the possibility of large-scale national immunization programs, so who needed local production?

More important were Mahoney's (and Gust's) doubts that the developing world, including Thailand, could successfully produce a high-technology vaccine. Plasma-derived vaccines were difficult enough, without even beginning to consider recombinant DNA ones. Mahoney feared a debacle. For Mahoney the problem with the vaccines was that they were to be injected into healthy babies, and thus the facilities would have to be first-rate.

They [vaccines] must be extremely high quality. . . . WHO has struggled to defend . . . [the] concept [of Good Manufacturing Practices (GMP)]. No developing country has a GMP facility! Not one! There are dozens that make vaccines. One could talk of accepting their limitations (dirty gowns, air-conditioning and temperature controls that are not perfect). . . . Accept the second classness of the developing world. That is not viable. . . . The developing world person does not accept it. . . . There have been a couple of disasters in the last couple of years. . . . This has led to the view that if the government wants local production—great—but they must build a GMP facility and they must build it, manage it, and have a regulatory authority that is meaningful. . . . Not a single developing country has a regulating authority that can protect quality. They must have the power to shut down the facility. . . . Most developing countries don't have the authority, or if they do, they don't have the technical ability to do quality control or inspection.[174]

There was a way out of this bind, according to Mahoney. If the Ministry of Education and Science (not the Ministry of Public Health) really wanted to produce vaccine, they could design a twenty-year-plan to develop that capacity: a high school program, a special college program in biologicals, chemical engineering, and so forth. They could develop a cadre of skilled workers, set up training institutes, and bring in experts on air-conditioning and other technical matters, and they could hope that in twenty years government salaries would grow fast enough (as in Korea) to keep the skilled people in government service.[175] Under the circumstances, however, the only positive use of the idea of local production had been to scare the big pharmaceutical companies into dropping their prices.

Mahoney believed that the problem for countries in the developing world stemmed directly from their overreliance on the public sector—both government and non-profit organizations—for getting things done. He felt that the public sector was inefficient even in the West, and all the more so outside of it. Non-profit organizations have many virtues, but suffer from a chronic lack of capital. Even the Dutch Red Cross, let alone the Thai Red Cross, lacked the money for a state-of-the-art factory. In developing countries an adequate supply of money is only available for the military. In other areas the government cannot afford to pay to keep good people. The public sector simply acts as a training ground for young people before they move over to the private sector at five times the salary.[176]

In Mahoney's opinion, the only positive function the government could play was in fostering competition in order to get the private sector to meet the needs of the people, rather than in trying to do so itself.[177] Idealistic individuals (and he was not without his share of such sentiments) may be attracted by the idea that private industry is full of materialists who do not care about human needs, but like it or not these "materialists" are the ones who can get the job done most efficiently. The trick is to motivate them, and to foster competition among them.

As far as the situation in Thailand went, Mahoney's declining enthusiasm was strongly affected by his use of the United Nations Industrial Development Organization's methodology for feasibility studies of technical production in the developing world. This methodology made creating a logical, step-by-step outline of what had to be done to set up local production possible, and it thus became clear to him that this was not a viable project. The domestic Thai market was too small to achieve the economies of scale that would bring the lowest prices. To get the larger market the Thais needed to export—but their neighbors were not interested. The Thai Red Cross would have to institute changes in its management procedures to become more like a private company if it wanted to succeed—and it was not willing to do so, even though it recognized that success depended on such changes.[178]

If it had been up to Mahoney, the Task Force would avoid involvement with the transfer of vaccine technology and would simply concentrate on getting the lowest possible price from the big pharmaceutical companies. But this was anathema to Maynard and Prince. Maynard felt that the private sector did not think in terms of the public good and of necessity left large numbers of human needs unmet. As long as it could find a profit in helping people it would, but when the profit was gone, the needs would be ignored. He was not opposed to a capitalist searching for profit per se, but the public sector was indispensable when private enterprise lost interest. The government simply had to produce and distribute the biologicals that the private sector did not.

Maynard saw the case of hepatitis B itself as illustrative of this very point. There was no indication that the drug companies initially were out to produce a low-cost vaccine for the majority of people. It took pressure outside the private sector (the Task Force) to forcefully redirect the companies' thinking toward the public sector so that the needs could be met.[179] The marketplace and profit motive by themselves did not, and could not, do it.[180]

Maynard also vehemently disagreed with Mahoney's view that the public sector was incapable of operating as efficiently and reliably as the private sector. The Europeans had proven that government could be effective: the Swiss railways are inferior to none. At the time, the public sector was falsely identified with the inefficient state enterprises of the communist regimes, and free market ideology was riding high, but, Maynard said, look at the effect of privatization of old-age homes and ask, "What does that tell you?"[181]

Maynard was especially incensed at the U.S. government's change in attitude toward the public sector under Reagan and Bush. USAID had always had a significant political component, but nevertheless had attempted to maintain a relatively unpolitical stance. Then it began to take the position, "To hell with national ownership; [to] hell with the public sector."[182] The issue became socialism versus capitalism, with no money available except for private enterprises. But, said Maynard, should all vaccines in the world be produced in a few Euro-American institutions? Should we not have technology transfer to developing areas—to both private and public organizations?[183]

These kinds of questions gave rise to raging discussions at Task Force meetings. Mahoney was the spokesman for the private sector: the marketplace and finance must decide, and one produces where it is best to produce—a free trade vision. He felt that PATH could harness private enterprise by using the legal concept of intellectual property rights: PATH would develop a product and license it to a private company, which would be required to supply the public sector at a certain price. Maynard said this was a fine idea as far as it went, but if the private sector developed the product itself—as it had with hepatitis B vaccine—then the method could not be used.[184]

In Mahoney's opinion, technology transfer only appeared to be useful when it was carried out successfully, which had not occurred in Thailand. But Maynard felt this view was not complex enough. He maintained that one can learn a lot even when transfer does not work in a particular country. Maynard believed a great deal had been learned simply from doing the feasibility study for Thailand. As far as Maynard was concerned, he and Prince had worked to make it happen in Thailand. They had tried to "knock heads together" in the Red Cross and the national government. In his words, they had attempted to

break the chicken and egg problem. The Thai Red Cross could not produce until the government said how much [vaccine] they needed. But the government wouldn't say what they would pay and guarantee to buy until the Red Cross told them they would produce it (and get the money to do it).[185]

It looked as if Task Force efforts had succeeded, but "at the last moment someone got to the government to say plasma vaccine was not safe."[186] There was tremendous hostility from Pasteur and other vaccine manufacturers to the Red Cross's producing vaccine, and Maynard felt that the government's fear may have come directly from drug company propaganda.[187] Nevertheless, Maynard thought, if Thailand were not fertile ground for technology transfer, some other place would be, perhaps Burma.

Nothing more clearly demonstrates Maynard and Prince's dedication to aiding developing countries to produce vaccine than their decision to get involved with the Burmese. One could not think of a more unlikely place for technology transfer than Burma. Burma's infrastructure was in a state of advanced decay, and they had trouble getting uncontaminated water in Rangoon, let alone doing high-technology production. But the Burmese needed hepatitis B vaccine desperately, and they lacked the foreign exchange to import the vaccine. Any chance to get hepatitis B vaccine to the Burmese children was better than no chance, or so Maynard and Prince felt.

Unity Despite Strong Differences of Philosophy in the Task Force

If Burma illustrates some Task Force members' unstinting dedication to local production, it also illuminates one of the group's most unusual qualities. While the Task Force was severely divided on the issue of public versus private sector and developing versus developed world vaccine production, no one let the disagreement destroy the unity of the group or create partisan discord within it. All views could be aired in the Task Force—with heat, energy, and emotion—and be accepted as legitimate.[188]

The Task Force did not founder on these conflicting views; rather, it thrived on the resulting "creative tension."[189] Maynard saw the disagreements not as liabilities but as indicators of the group's basic strength. The socialistic bias of men like himself, Prince, and Gust counterbalanced the pro-private sector bias of Mahoney. The free expression of competing views, vehemently and cogently presented, served to protect the group from veering too far to the left or the right. It helped them to steer a middle course and thus maintain the delicate balance between practicality and idealism that was necessary for their survival in international health politics.[190] As Prince saw it:

A key element of the success of the Task Force is an artful mixture of different degrees of scientific dreamer personalities and politically savvy personalities . . . [who are] doers. All have a little of each to get along [together] but all have different degrees of this mix. Rich [Mahoney] is 70% doer and 30% dreamer. Gust is 70% political and Maynard is very political—but of course also a dreamer. I am less political than [they are, more of a dreamer].[191]

The Task Force appreciated the importance of both dreamers and doers and was tolerant of the conflicts these individuals constantly generated.

Most important, everyone was willing to subordinate his or her ideological position and ego to the common goal of making the Task Force effective. Where other groups would have broken apart and self-destructed, or forced a stultifying uniformity of views on the membership, the Task Force was energized, and protected, by the conflicting views its members generated.[192]

Many members felt the Burmese venture was doomed to failure. They would not endorse it as an official Task Force project, but they respected Maynard and Prince's desire to be involved, and they gave them the freedom to work for it:

[Thus] Fred [Prince] and I [Maynard] are consultants [to the South East Asian Regional Office of WHO (SEARO)-sponsored project. It is] not a Task Force activity per se. It isn't ours, but it is a distinction without a difference. In fact the same sort of work is being done using Task Force members.[193]

In Mahoney's eyes, the Task Force, if it were to take a vote on Burma, would not go forward. But if the project were going to be done anyway with United Nations money, "we would make it less than an unmitigated disaster."[194] The Task Force could and did stretch to accommodate both sides of the issue.

Thus, the Thai technology transfer issue brought to the surface many of the conflicting beliefs and attitudes found among Task Force members. While the issue strained the cohesion of the group, it did not break the Task Force, but rather once again demonstrated the strength to which tolerance of diversity and conflict give rise.

Conclusions

As we look back on the activities of the Task Force in Thailand, certain aspects of its experience stand out. Of key importance is that successful intervention in a developing country requires concern with and intimate knowledge of the local political, social, and scientific scene. One cannot positively affect conditions in a country such as Thailand by blundering in like a Western bull in an Asian china shop. The Task Force had to know and respect the established way of doing things and not impose its rules or values on the people with whom it dealt. The Task Force, using PATH's experience and contacts, was able to function at a comparatively sophisticated level in the game of Thai power politics. It skillfully used the groups that existed in Bangkok and, just as importantly, allowed itself to be used by them in ways that furthered the goal of fighting the hepatitis B epidemic. The Task Force functioned more as a catalyst than a creator of the Thai national effort, which, given the already existing high level of interest in hepatitis B, was exactly what the situation demanded.

Given the incredible number of people and groups that wanted to be involved in any project the Task Force financed, the most important thing for the organization to do was to elicit as much information from each of the potential collaborators and separate the truth from the rumors and false claims. What proved especially difficult was the myriad of personal interconnections among the different factions as they sometimes competed and sometimes cooperated on a host of different projects. The Task Force virtually had to keep a scorecard to know who was politically "in" or "out" at any given moment.

The Task Force's greatest success came from its detailed knowledge of the sociopolitical situation in Thailand, and its greatest failure came from a (perhaps unavoidable) miscalculation of the power of one of its allies. The lesson from Thailand is that success for a determined activist group such as the Task Force comes only from a thorough mastery of the details on the ground. Local political situations place definite limitations on what an outside group can accomplish. In Thailand rivalries and hidden interests existed which no foreigners (and few natives) could fully understand or overcome.

Notes

1. Memo by Henry Wilde to Richard Mahoney, March 6, 1985, talking about the view of the Section Chief of the Rabies Control Division, Thailand.

2. See John Girling, *Thailand: Society and Politics* (Ithaca, N.Y.: Cornell University Press, 1981). Traditionally in Thailand economic activity was dominated by the ethnic Chinese, with Thai energies going into the bureaucracy. In the 1950s the government established Thai state enterprises as a source of revenue for the government, as a means for leading bureaucrats to get private gain, and as a way for Thais to develop their entrepreneurship. In addition, in response to the Chinese economic challenge, they established semi-official Thai trading ventures, based on patron–client lines. By the late 1950s the government moved from competing with the Chinese enterprises to instead attempting to give support to the entire economy; in turn, the Chinese moved to assimilate themselves into Thai society and develop business-bureaucratic cooperation along clique lines. Increasingly, a large part of the bureaucratic elite came from Chinese trading families or the Chinese in general. As time went on government intervention in the economy became better organized and refined as a result of the work of Thai technocrats who were largely Western-trained financial experts, managers, planners, and economists. These experts were given considerable power within their spheres of competence, but only as long as they accepted the general bureaucratic polity system. The increasing aim of the technocrats within the bureaucracy was to encourage free market forces and discourage state intervention—especially on the grounds of welfare. While there has been a significant merger of the bureaucracy and the entrepreneurial groups, the patronage system still distorts the market, according to Girling, because "by favoring one enterprise rather than another for reasons of personal advantage (instead of reasons of cost, quality, or efficiency) it distorts or impedes economic growth," as well as leads to corruption (pp. 72–83, 143, 185).

3. Memo by Mahoney to Thai File, Asian trip #1, November 1, 1984.

4. Ibid.

5. The status of Crown Princess indicates that she is eligible to inherit the throne.

6. Thai names are written in a fashion similar to Western names: first name,

then surname. But unlike in the West, when a person is addressed or referred to, a man is called by his first name, not his surname. Thus Dr. Kachorn Pranich is called Dr. Kachorn. Many foreigners do not realize this and assume that Kachorn is the last name. It is common in PATH documents for Thai last names to be ignored. The fact that there are many people called "Dr. Kachorn" can be quite confusing unless one knows the organization to which they are attached.

7. Memo by Mahoney to Thai File, Asian trip #5, November 1, 1984.

8. Ibid. He also owned a company "which imports and distributes medical equipment, undertakes the construction of radio and television transmitting towers and owns a private hospital" (memo by Mahoney to Thai File, Asian trip #13, November 6, 1984).

9. Memo by Mahoney to Thai File, Asian trip #6, November 1, 1984.

10. Memo by Mahoney to Thai File, Asian trip #25, November 1, 1984.

11. Memo by Mahoney to Gordon W. Perkin, President of PATH, December 13, 1984, discussing the meeting with Scott Halstead of the Rockefeller Foundation.

12. Memo by Mahoney to Thai File, Asian trip #13, November 6, 1984.

13. Letter from T. Pangsrivongse of B. L. Hua and Co. to Mahoney, May 16, 1985.

14. Ibid.

15. Memo by Henry Wilde to Mahoney, October 26, 1985; interview with Wilde, January 30, 1992.

16. Memo by Mahoney to Henry Wilde, October 17, 1985.

17. Memo by Wilde to Mahoney, Asian trip #33, March 6, 1985.

18. Ibid., quoting a high government official.

19. Memo by Wilde to Mahoney, May 23, 1985, concerning talks with Prof. Natth.

20. Ibid.

21. Ibid.; memo by Wilde to Mahoney, June 13, 1985, concerning talks with Prof. Natth.

22. Memo by Wilde to Mahoney, June 12, 1985.

23. Ibid. Natth is talking specifically about the technological transfer of diagnostics rather than vaccine production, but his views are consistent with it.

24. Memo by Wilde to Mahoney, May 23, 1985. On the memo is handwritten the words "Do not final, put 'not finalled' on the comments section."

25. Memo by Mahoney to Wilde, June 11, 1985.

26. Ibid.

27. Memo by Wilde to Mahoney, June 13, 1985.

28. Natth believed that PATH and the Task Force became involved with the Red Cross primarily because of Wilde's contacts there, but such is not the case. Memos in the PATH files also show that Natth did not have a consistent anti-technology transfer position over time, but rather changed back and forth on the issue.

29. Memo by Mongkol to Mahoney, July 15, 1985.

30. Memo by Mahoney to Hepatitis B File, August 15, 1985, concerning the talk with Maynard on August 9, 1985.

31. Ibid.

32. Memo by Wilde to Mahoney, October 22, 1985.

33. Memo by Wilde to Mahoney, June 25, 1985, concerning the talk with Praphan; memo by Wilde to Mahoney, October 22, 1985. Most of the PATH

material discusses what is going on in the Red Cross Institute because Wilde was associated with it. The Institute was important in the technology transfer issue, but the part of the Red Cross actually directly concerned with potential manufacture was the National Blood Center, which owned the blood. The Institute and Blood Center had separate staffs and were rivals of each other. It was the National Blood Center that had the strongest ties to the Dutch; the Institute was primarily concerned with using the vaccine in its clinics (memo by Wilde, December 17, 1986).

34. Memo by Mahoney to Hepatitis B File, October 2, 1985.

35. Memo by Mahoney to Wilde, October 17, 1985.

36. Ibid.

37. Memo by Wilde to Mahoney, October 25, 1985.

38. Ibid.

39. Memo by Wilde to Hepatitis B File, May 21, 1986, concerning the meeting with Prof. W. G. Van Aken. The quotation marks are in the original.

40. Memo by Wilde to Mahoney, October 26, 1985.

41. Ibid.

42. Memo by Wilde to Mahoney, #5, concerning the Dutch Red Cross/ Central Laboratory meeting on January 14, 1986, with Prof. Van Aken and Mr. Arie Langstraat.

43. Ibid.

44. Ibid.

45. Interview with Anton Widjaya, January 21, 1992, where he made this assessment of the Indonesian Red Cross.

46. Memos by Mahoney to Health Link File, May 5, 1986; April 19, 1986.

47. Memo by Wilde to Hepatitis B File, May 9, 1986.

48. Ibid.

49. Memo by Wilde to Mahoney, March 6, 1986; memo by Wilde to Hepatitis B File, March 9, 1986.

50. Memo by Wilde to Hepatitis B File, May 12, 1986, concerning the meeting with S. J. Lee of Cheil. A number of Thais, including Drs. Supawat, Praphan, and Somsak (of the Ministry of Public Health), were present.

51. Ibid.

52. Memo by Wilde to Hepatitis B File, October 24, 1986, concerning the visit to Reesink of the Dutch Red Cross.

53. Memo by Wilde to Hepatitis B File, May 21, 1986.

54. Ibid.

55. Memo by Mahoney, #1, June 4, 1986, dealing with the May 29–30, 1986, meeting to implement the new hepatitis B task force.

56. Memo by Mahoney to Hepatitis B File, May 6, 1986, dealing with Mahoney's April 23, 1986, trip to Seoul, Korea.

57. Letter from Prince to Wilde, July 16, 1986.

58. Memo by Wilde, January 21, 1987.

59. Memo by Wilde, December 13, 1986.

60. Memo by Wilde, December 17, 1986.

61. Memo by Wilde, February 17, 1986.

62. Ibid.

63. Memo by Mahoney, #1, February 4, 1987, reporting on the January 13, 1987, meeting; also memo by Mahoney, #2, February 4, 1987. After hearing Mr. Arie Langstraat's pessimism about the situation, Mahoney was moved to "state . . . as strongly as possible my personal view that it would be unfortunate

if the [Dutch Red Cross] . . . were to cease production of hepatitis B vaccine as seemed likely from the conversation."

64. Memo by Wilde to Mahoney, #5, February 4, 1986, concerning the meeting with the Dutch Red Cross on January 14, 1986.

65. Memo by Wilde to Hepatitis B File, March 31, 1987, concerning the telephone conversation with Langstraat of the Dutch Red Cross.

66. According to Prof. Van Aken, the actual withdrawal of the Dutch from hepatitis B manufacturing had more to do with the "devastating . . . collapse of prices" which the Task Force's activities had brought about, "not the poor lot of vaccine." However, the price problem was compounded by the fact that the recombinant DNA vaccine was about to come out, and the Dutch Red Cross's internal market (where high prices were still possible) was already very small because the national health insurance authorities refused to pay for vaccine for homosexuals and intravenous drug users, the two largest high-risk groups in the Netherlands. He did not emphasize problems with WHO standards, bad publicity, or any other reasons. I was surprised to find him very guarded and wary during the interview, as if he were very concerned not to offend important people or groups. As a result, when I found that his recollection of the situation in 1986–87 conflicted with PATH documents from that period, I made the judgment that the documents were more reliable. This was especially true of what he said about the setting of WHO biological standards for hepatitis B vaccines, which he defended (interview with Van Aken, June 2, 1992).

67. Memo by Prince to Mahoney, April 4, 1987.

68. Memo by Donald Douglas to Hepatitis B File, December 19, 1986.

69. Memo by Wilde to Hepatitis B File, December 18, 1986.

70. Ibid.

71. Memo by Donald Douglas to Hepatitis B File, December 19, 1986.

72. Ibid.

73. Memo by Wilde to Hepatitis B File, December 18, 1986.

74. Memo by Douglas to Hepatitis B File, December 19, 1986.

75. Ibid.

76. Ibid.

77. Ibid.

78. Ibid.

79. Documents do not provide a last name.

80. Memo by Wilde to Hepatitis B File, December 21, 1986.

81. Memo by Mahoney, February 3, 1987, concerning the Amsterdam/Bangkok trip, #5.

82. Memo by Mahoney, February 3, 1987, concerning the Amsterdam/Bangkok trip, #13.

83. Memo by Mahoney, February 3, 1987, concerning the Amsterdam/Bangkok trip, #12. Princess Chulakorn was the second princess of the royal family.

84. The existence of so many task forces, and such widespread interest in hepatitis B, made Thailand a very fertile place for the International Task Force to establish a model program. But it was also clear that to move from interest and discussion to actual action required a dynamic push—one provided by the International Task Force.

85. Richard Mahoney, February 3, 1987, Amsterdam/Bangkok trip, #16.

86. Memo by Douglas to Hepatitis B File, March 31, 1987, concerning meetings on February 25–27, 1987.

87. Ibid.

88. Ibid.

89. Ibid.

90. Interview with Supamit, January 31, 1992, but without any negative interpretation of its significance.

91. "A Proposal to the James S. McDonnell Foundation, Support of the International Task Force on Hepatitis B Immunization," July 1989, submitted by PATH.

92. "A Model Immunization Program for Hepatitis B Vaccine in Thailand— Preliminary Protocol," Draft, August 1987.

93. Interview with Supamit, January 31, 1992.

94. Ibid.

95. Interview with Douglas, January 27, 1992.

96. Interview with Wilde, January 30, 1992.

97. Interview with Supamit, January 31, 1992.

98. Interview with Douglas, January 27, 1992.

99. Discussed at the Task Force meeting in Houston, April 3–4, 1990. The Task Force became involved with the Jordan model program after Dr. Ala Toukan of Jordan joined the group. He had designed the project.

100. Interview with Douglas, January 27, 1992.

101. Interview with Supamit, January 31, 1992.

102. Interview with Natth, January 31, 1992.

103. Ibid.

104. Interview with Supamit, January 31, 1992.

105. Ibid.

106. Ibid.

107. Interview with Douglas, February 28, 1992.

108. Memo by Yuenyong Dao-Chaeng to Douglas, May 17, 1988, concerning the meeting on the Launching Ceremony with the Ministry of Public Health Team.

109. March 1991. Appendix 1: Executive summary: Information, Education and Communication Evaluation of Thailand's Hepatitis B Immunization model program. "1990 Annual Narrative and Financial Report to the James S. McDonnell Foundation from the International Task Force on Hepatitis B Immunization."

110. Interview with Douglas, January 28, 1992.

111. "1990 Annual Narrative."

112. Ibid.

113. Ibid.

114. Interview with Douglas, January 26, 1992.

115. Ibid.

116. March 1991. Executive summary, "1990 Annual Narrative and Financial Report to the McDonnell Foundation from the International Task Force."

117. Ibid.

118. Interview with Supamit, January 31, 1992.

119. Discussion at Task Force meeting in Houston, April 3–4, 1990.

120. Interview with Maynard, September 11, 1991; interview with Supamit, January 31, 1992.

121. "Hepatitis B Vaccine for Use in the Model Immunization Program," a report of the International Task Force on Hepatitis B Immunization to the Thai Ministry of Public Health and the Thai Red Cross Society, September 1987.

122. Interview with Prayura, January 31, 1992.

123. Not only the Thais felt this way. In a letter to Dr. G. Duraisamy, Director of the National Blood Transfusion Service of Malaysia, dated June 6, 1988, Maynard had to respond to his concern about the Japanese and Korean plasma-derived vaccines. Duraisamy had asked why these vaccines were not on sale in the United States, and Maynard replied, "There is the widespread impression that if certain pharmaceuticals and biologics are not licensed in the United States or Britain, they must be inferior. Nothing could be farther from the truth. . . . It is because . . . a decision to seek licensure in a particular country is based also upon a marketing opinion regarding whether the expense and complications involved in seeking licensure are worth the anticipated share of market to be secured," not just quality considerations. He could also have said that the U.S. Food and Drug Administration regulations are used to discourage foreign manufacturers from competing in the United States, and that the Americans are irrational in their fear of plasma-derived vaccines, though making the last point would have been counterproductive.

124. "Hepatitis B Vaccine for Use in the Model Immunization Program." The claim of Dutch involvement was clearly misleading.

125. Ibid.

126. Donald Douglas to Mahoney, April 20, 1989.

127. Donald Douglas to Mahoney, August 11, 1989, includes "a summary" of Dr. Praphan's study under the title "Comparative Study of the Anti-HBs and Anti-PRE S2 Response to Four Plasma-derived Hepatitis B Vaccines in Thai Young Adults."

128. Memo by Douglas to Maynard et al., April 20, 1989.

129. Interview with Douglas, January 27, 1992. Cheil vaccine could be imported without registration only as long as importation was done through the Thai Red Cross, which had special rights that freed it from the normal Food and Drug Administration and other requirements.

130. Letter from Mahoney to Shin, May 4, 1989.

131. Interview with Douglas, January 27, 1992.

132. Interview with Dr. Praphan Panpark, Chulalongkorn University and Red Cross Institute, January 31, 1992; memo from Mahoney to Douglas and Maynard, October 30, 1989.

133. Interview with Prince, January 29, 1991; interview with Maynard, June 18, 1991. It is probable that they would also agree with Ward Morehouse, President of the Council on International and Public Affairs, who wrote "The harsh reality is that a country which is almost entirely dependent on external sources for vital health care needs is just as vulnerable as one that is dependent on [outside sources] . . . for essential foodstuffs. . . . [I]f developing countries were to band together and unilaterally renounce some or all of their external debt," they would be vulnerable to having vaccine, insulin, and other imported pharmaceuticals shut off ("Strengthening Developing Country Capacity for Meeting Their Own Health Care Needs: The Production of 'Orphan Vaccines,'" a discussion paper, Draft, February 15, 1990, attached to a letter to Maynard, asking for his critical comments).

134. Miriam Ryan, "Hepatitis B Vaccine Contract Goes to Untested Product," *Nature,* 329 (1987): 6. The journal issued a retraction a couple of weeks later ("Hepatitis B: Correction," *Nature* 329 (1987): 278.

135. Ryan, "Hepatitis B Vaccine Contract," 6.

136. "The Price Is Right: Cheap Hepatitis Vaccine Offers Immunization

Breakthrough," *Far East Review* (October 10, 1989). (An English translation of this article is in the Task Force files. The language and place of origin is not stated.)

137. Interview with Maynard, July 7, 1993.

138. "A Proposal to the James S. McDonnell Foundation, Support of the International Task Force on Hepatitis B Immunization," July 1989, submitted by PATH.

139. Memo by Mahoney to Douglas, March 23, 1989.

140. Ibid.

141. Memo by Mahoney to Douglas, March 26, 1989.

142. Memo by Wilde to Hepatitis B File, May 9, 1986, concerning the discussion with Praphan. Praphan seems to have been talking specifically about production of vaccine, not processing per se, but his views seem to encompass both equally well.

143. Supawat actually felt that neither the National Blood Center nor anyone else in Thailand had much chance of success for a variety of reasons, and by this point Wilde agreed with that negative assessment: "They do not have the staff that would have the time, motivation and perseverance to follow through in the long run. It is too complex a project for amateurs and part-time workers" (memo by Wilde to Mahoney, November 16, 1988).

144. Memo by Douglas to Mahoney, April 18, 1989, concerning the meeting with Supamit at the Red Cross.

145. Memo by Mahoney to Douglas, May 31, 1989.

146. Memo by Mahoney to Douglas, May 26, 1989.

147. Ibid.

148. "Report and Recommendations to the Thai Red Cross Society on the Technology Transfer for Hepatitis B Vaccine Production," submitted by the International Task Force on Hepatitis B Immunization, August 1989.

149. Ibid.

150. Letter by Mahoney to Mr. H. K. Kim, Managing Director of Cheil, June 29, 1989.

151. Memo by Mahoney to Douglas, March 23, 1989.

152. Memo by Mahoney to Maynard, October 26, 1989.

153. Ibid.

154. Memo by PATH-Thailand to PATH-Seattle, October 15, 1989.

155. Ibid.

156. Memo by Mahoney to Maynard, October 26, 1989.

157. Ibid.

158. Memo by Douglas to Mahoney, December 29, 1989.

159. Memo by Mahoney to Douglas, February 8, 1990.

160. Interview with a high-ranking Thai official who wished to remain anonymous.

161. Interview with Prayura, Deputy Director of the Thai Communicable Disease Control Division, January 31, 1992.

162. Memo by Wilde to Hepatitis B File, May 9, 1986. Emphasis added.

163. Ibid.

164. Interview with Prayura, January 31, 1992.

165. Interview with Natth, January 31, 1992.

166. Interview with Prayura, January 31, 1992.

167. Interview with Supamit, January 31, 1992.

168. Interview with Natth, January 31, 1992.

169. Interview with Praphan, January 31, 1992.

170. Interview with Wilde, January 30, 1991.

171. Interview with Maynard, June 6, 1992.

172. Interview with Prince, March 27, 1991.

173. Draft of the "Minutes of the Annual Meeting of the International Task Force on Hepatitis B Immunization," Houston, Texas, April 3–4, 1990.

174. Interview with Mahoney, June 20, 1991. According to Mahoney, Korea is for most purposes a developed country.

175. Ibid.

176. Interview with Mahoney, April 29, 1991.

177. Ibid.

178. Ibid.

179. Interview with Maynard, June 18, 1991.

180. This view is supported by Dr. Anthony Robbins, a highly knowledgeable observer of the vaccine field. He says hepatitis B vaccine investment decisions were primarily made for the industrial world market and its high prices. He asks, "Would they have gone into production [at all] without an industrial world market base?" He does not believe so. Commercial firms look to market priorities. He, like Maynard and Prince, asks "Is the increasing dominance of vaccine production by commercial firms irreconcilable with the public health goals of the developing world?" He answers, "Yes." (He is also very laudatory about the work of the Task Force.) See Anthony Robbins, M.D., and Phyllis Freeman, J.D., "Can We Expedite the Fruits of Vaccine Research?" *7th Session of the WHO Scientific Advisory Group of Experts* (SAGE)(WHO) June 25–27, 1990, agenda item 13, pp. 1–17.

181. Interview with Maynard, June 18, 1991.

182. Interview with Maynard, June 17, 1991.

183. Ibid.

184. Interview with Maynard, June 18, 1991.

185. Interview with Maynard, June 19, 1991.

186. Ibid.

187. Ibid.

188. Interview with Prince, January 29, 1991. Prince put the situation this way: "It is very important to have freewheeling discussions. Then be persuaded, back down, realize one's position is bullshit. What is published later is the consensus. The earlier positions often are stupid, and would embarrass people."

189. Interview with Maynard, June 17, 1991.

190. Interview with Maynard, June 19, 1991.

191. Interview with Prince, January 29, 1991.

192. Interview with Maynard, June 19, 1991.

193. Interview with Maynard, January 25, 1991.

194. Interview with Mahoney, June 20, 1991.

Chapter 5
The Task Force and WHO: Conflict and Cooperation

As important as the model projects in Thailand and Indonesia were for the International Task Force on Hepatitis B Immunization, the ultimate fate of its efforts would be determined on a different stage. The goal of universal hepatitis B immunization could not be achieved without the active support of the World Health Organization (WHO) and its Expanded Programme on Immunization (EPI). It was in Geneva that the Task Force would either win or lose its battle.

This chapter looks closely at the constantly changing relationship between the Task Force and WHO as they struggled to reach some form of mutual accommodation. Their often difficult association was manifested in places as far-flung as China, Africa, the Philippines, the Caribbean, and Europe.

The Task Force played a role in the continuing conflict among pharmaceutical companies vying for a larger share of the hepatitis B vaccine market, and the fight played itself out in WHO meetings. Whether the Task Force was dealing with WHO or hostile drug companies, its primary goal was not to defeat those who opposed it but rather to deal first with their concerns and then win them over as allies.

The Task Force and WHO: Love and Hate

The relationship between the Task Force and WHO resembled a tumultuous marriage: couldn't live together, couldn't live apart. Counseling the couple required much tact and great delicacy. At first glance the two organizations appeared made for each other. In the eyes of James Maynard and Ian Gust, the International Task Force on Hepatitis B Immunization developed at least in part as a logical outgrowth of WHO's Western Pacific Regional Office (WPRO) Task Force on Hepatitis B, to which they were major contributors. In addition, Maynard and R. Palmer Beasley were two of WHO-Geneva's main consulting experts for hepatitis problems worldwide, and many of the International Task Force's members were prominent in the Technical Advisory Groups (TAGs) and Global Advisory Groups (GAGs) that were the major channels through which WHO created health policy. Right from the start of the Task Force, people like Maynard wore two hats, that of the Task Force and that of the World Health Organization, a situation that served to enhance the prestige of the young organization for officials in Thailand, Indonesia, and elsewhere. Later, both the Task Force and the Program for Appropriate Technology in Health (PATH) were jointly awarded coveted status as a WHO Collaborating Centre for Hepatitis B Vaccination. This was an exceptional designation for such a private group, since that status was usually reserved for government facilities or universities. In fact, there was no precedent for this status being conferred on a non-governmental organization. It had to be created de novo for the Task Force and PATH.[1]

In a very real sense people like Maynard could say "the World Health Organization, c'est moi!" and that reality went far toward muting and controlling the conflicts that arose between the Task Force and WHO. Nevertheless, discord abounded, and substantial effort was required to contain and counteract it. Conflict was unavoidably built into their relationship as a result of the vast scope of the WHO mandate. WHO had as its responsibility the protection and improvement of the health of mankind, but it lacked the funds and staff to fulfill its all-inclusive mission. A political problem would inevitably arise if some other group entered the health arena and attempted to deal with a disease that fell under WHO's general mandate. Such presumption threatened a significant loss of face for the organization.

Clearly, many in the WHO bureaucracy felt insulted by the appearance on the scene of these self-appointed experts, but this was not a uniform response, and some important officials expressed pleasure at the prospect of getting help in an area where they lacked resources. Nevertheless, the predominant response at WHO did not involve putting the official goal of promoting health above organizational or personal ego considerations (any more than it would have elsewhere).[2]

Maynard and Gust, both deeply committed to WHO, were quite understanding and tolerant of the conflict. They were convinced that, with a little diplomacy and tact, the key figures at WHO could be won over. It was important that the Task Force avoid appearing as a competitor; instead, it had to emphasize its supportive role.

Maynard was quite aware that avoiding confrontation would be exceptionally difficult. He put the problem this way:

For twenty years I have had a close relationship with WHO. . . . Gust also has had [it]. . . . WHO initiates action or sends us on expeditions to a country. WHO has a masterplan—we helped develop it but as their advisors. The question of who is leading who is not a problem. The Task Force is a newcomer. We say we want to work with and for WHO. But we are developing our own agenda. . . . [O]ur flexibility means we can act when others can't act. But what we do will give the appearance that we are leading, not following. . . . Some in WHO will adjust [and say] "we will follow." Others will not adjust; they are resentful of Task Force initiative.[3]

In Maynard's view, one simply had to make every effort to relieve the tensions that developed.

Members of the Task Force other than Maynard and Gust felt less charitable. They saw WHO as a highly politicized, bureaucratic maze that engaged in endless talk and accomplished very little. They would probably agree with the scathing assessment made by Kenneth Warren, M.D., ex-Director of the Health Science Division of the Rockefeller Foundation:

WHO thinks it owns everything in health. If anyone from outside gets involved and invades their turf they rally round the covered wagon. They are very defensive and hostile. . . . Everyone kisses asses at WHO—they think they need it. Ninety percent of those at work at WHO are hacks, concerned only with self-aggrandizement; they have ten percent very talented people [and only] if you find them can you get things done.[4]

But even those who saw WHO in such an unflattering light realized that cooperating with WHO was fundamental to the success of their mission, and they were supportive of Maynard-style diplomacy. The WHO staff also ultimately had to deal with the fact that if they wanted to achieve anything in the fight against hepatitis B they had to cooperate with the Task Force, regardless of their own feelings.

WHO and the Task Force in China: Conflict and Reconciliation

A perfect example of the cooperation and conflict that co-existed in the relationship between the two organizations occurred in the People's Republic of China. The transfer of hepatitis B vaccine technology to China by the WPRO Hepatitis Task Force constituted the group's crowning achievement, and both Gust and Maynard had been intimately involved in that process. However, the goal of universal vaccination, or even large-scale production, had not been achieved. The International Task Force saw a need for more work in China and felt there was a role for it to play in promoting the integration of hepatitis B

into the Chinese EPI and helping to lower the vaccine price by intro-
ducing more efficient production methods. As a result of discussions
with the Chinese government, a "decision was made to recognize the
[International] Task Force as an entity with the exact same credentials
as WHO."[5] It was an unexpected and unrequested coup; the consequences for the Task Force's prestige were immense. As Maynard put
it, "Suddenly we were dealt with on the same level as the World Health
Organization."[6] The leaders of WPRO, as the regional representatives
of WHO, were enraged. This constituted a terrible loss of face—a
situation magnified by the fact that WPRO was led by Drs. Nakajima
Hiroshi and Umenai Takusai, both Japanese nationals, for whom matters of prestige had great importance.

The situation was particularly aggravating to Nakajima (later the
Director-General of WHO-Geneva), who prided himself on having
personally opened China to WHO activities, only to find someone
trespassing on his turf. He asked Maynard to meet with him and
Umenai in September 1987 in Beijing, where Maynard found two very
enraged WPRO leaders. In Maynard's account, Umenai angrily demanded to know, "What right does the Task Force have to be in China
[at all]." Fortunately, Eric Goon, head of WPRO's local office in China
and a friend of the Task Force, was also present. Goon "charged to
their defense," telling Nakajima that the Task Force's only goal was to
help and that the decision to give the Task Force such a high status was
one made entirely by the Chinese. With Nakajima somewhat appeased,
Maynard "tried to soothe the waters" by saying that while the Task
Force would not agree to seek WPRO approval for everything they did
in China, WPRO could and should "coopt us, use us, and take the
credit" for any good that was accomplished.[7]

During the meeting the participants agreed that the Task Force and
WHO would co-sponsor a pilot project in Long An County to demonstrate the feasibility of integrating hepatitis B immunization into the
Chinese EPI. Maynard came away from the meeting quite satisfied that
real progress had been achieved.[8]

The Long An County project had been suggested in 1986 when
WHO experts had visited China and decided that a rural model program should be started there. At WPRO's request the model program
had been designed by one of those experts—James Maynard.[9] Now,
after the Beijing meeting, the Task Force had for almost all intents and
purposes been given that model program as its own project. Later, the
agreement between the two organizations was explained to the Chinese Minister of Health as a simple cooperative venture: "A project
proposal was developed [by WPRO], which WHO has [now] given to
the Task Force with a request for assistance in funding and monitor-

ing."[10] WHO had transferred the project because WPRO could not locate funding for the project and felt the Task Force could.[11]

In addition to the model project in Long An County, the Task Force became involved in upgrading Chinese local hepatitis B vaccine production. The Task Force personnel believed the technology transfer that WPRO had promoted, while admirable, used a methodology that was not capable of meeting China's vast needs. Rather, they contended that the flash heating-inactivation procedure used by the New York Blood Center was many times more efficient and would radically raise Chinese vaccine productivity—which was a vital goal.[12] Although the Chinese wanted to import recombinant DNA vaccine technology, the Task Force recommended that that goal be put aside for the time being.

The fact that Maynard had designed the Long An County project as a WHO consultant and then inherited it as a Task Force leader lies very much at the core of the complex relationship between the two organizations. As the project proceeded both Maynard and Beasley acted as monitors and consultants,[13] and they served simultaneously as Task Force and WHO/WPRO representatives in those capacities. In a fundamental way WHO could not make war on the Task Force without doing battle with itself, and this provided essential protection for the newly formed organization.

The Long An County model was in many respects a success for both the Task Force and China, proving that even in one of the poorest and most underdeveloped rural areas in China integration of hepatitis B into the EPI was possible. The project was able to significantly lower the carrier rate among children in the county. A major finding of the studies done of Long An County also strongly suggested that the hepatitis B vaccine was sufficiently stable under normal temperature conditions and that it could be used beyond the cold chain. The term *cold chain* refers to the requirement that vaccines be kept at a constant low temperature from manufacture to delivery—a process which entails significant expensive and assiduous care. The lack of cooling apparatus (and the power to run it) in rural areas presented a monumental problem for the administration of EPI vaccines throughout the world. It certainly militated against early vaccination in the home or rural hamlet because the vaccine could be kept cold only in selected locations. Now it appeared that hepatitis B vaccine could be kept unrefrigerated for long periods even in remote villages, which would make early vaccination a much more practical affair.[14]

The China project, like those in Indonesia and Thailand, was not without its disappointments, especially in regard to local production of vaccine. The Task Force (with WHO's blessing) believed that high-efficiency plasma vaccines were best suited for China as well as the rest of the developing world. The capital expense required to produce recombinant DNA vaccine was tremendous compared with that for plasma, and the vaccine was no better.[15] The Task Force persisted in recommending that the Chinese upgrade their plasma vaccine facilities and not go forward with recombinant DNA technology transfer. This recommendation was especially important because the conditions they found at the Chinese vaccine facilities were quite appalling.[16] But the Chinese could not resist the prestige of producing recombinant DNA and reached an agreement with Merck to establish the process in China. In the eyes of the Task Force and a minority of Chinese officials, this was a tragic mistake. To make matters worse, the Chinese, as part of their movement to a market-oriented economy, had made hepatitis B vaccine available on the basis of ability to pay. The price, while affordable for urban dwellers, was too expensive for the majority of rural inhabitants. As a result, even though production was insufficient for the population's needs, undistributed vaccine sat on warehouse shelves. Now, with the additional capital expenses for the production of recombinant DNA vaccine, the price would rise rather than fall. (Radical critics of "vertical" high-technology programs often see capitalism and Western indoctrination as the malignant forces behind such ambitious programs, but China's attitude toward recombinant DNA vaccine production does not support such a view.)

While the Task Force strongly opposed recombinant DNA production, it was willing to be involved in technology transfer and vaccine production in order to insure that the process was done as safely and efficiently as possible, if the Chinese insisted upon going forward with it. The Task Force prided itself on its nondogmatic flexibility. Ultimately, the decision to produce or not produce vaccine—either the plasma or recombinant DNA variety—was a local governmental responsibility, and the Task Force accepted and respected that fact. Maynard and Prince, who felt committed to technology transfer because of their commitment to the ideal of Third World independence from Western control, were particularly sensitive to the need for respecting the government's wishes.

The Problem of Setting Reasonable Vaccine Standards at WHO

The Task Force was also deeply concerned about and involved with WHO's activities in setting vaccine production standards. One of the biggest problems the Task Force faced in convincing developing countries such as Thailand to embrace the Cheil vaccine and its inexpensive methodology was Cheil's failure to meet the production guidelines set down by WHO. (This shortcoming also plagued the Korean Green Cross Corporation [KGCC], the Dutch Red Cross, and the more prestigious French Pasteur Vaccins.)

When the Task Force was organized, the existing WHO standards for vaccines were exceptionally rigorous—many people considered them unreasonably so—and the suspicion existed that the inability of most vaccine manufacturers to meet those standards was not coincidental. Alfred Prince had been present at the original Biological Standards meeting designed to establish WHO's recommendations for minimum requirements for plasma-derived vaccines.[17] No country was obliged to follow WHO's advice, but the recommendations constituted the international benchmark against which vaccines would be measured.[18] Prince[19] was "not very political" or experienced with the workings of WHO, and, as he put it, "I was so naive about WHO I did not know we were writing requirements." The suggested regulations that came out of the meeting were basically "you must make it the way Merck does." Prince felt that the meeting was dominated by Dr. Maurice Hilleman, who Prince found an "overpowering personality." Hilleman was an internationally respected scientist and the man most responsible for creating a commercially viable hepatitis B vaccine—for Merck, which employed him. He received overwhelming support for his views from the other scientists, some of whom, Prince believed, were themselves consultants to Merck.

One of the key aspects of the requirements involved a level of purity for the vaccine that was only achievable by using the process Merck employed. From Prince's standpoint the level of purity obtained by that process was not vital, but the standard constituted "a very clever maneuver because only Merck would have a WHO approved vaccine."[20] Prince knew that the New York Blood Center vaccine could never meet those requirements; he argued against them, but to no avail. Not coincidentally, in Prince's opinion, the Pasteur vaccine was also shut out by the standards adopted. Frank Perkins, the Chief of Biologicals, played an important role in creating the standard, and he not only believed that the developing world lacked the ability to produce acceptable vaccines, he also was skeptical of the French company's capabilities. (Ian Gust saw the meeting as at least in part a fight between "the English-speaking . . . [and] the non-English speaking" scientists, with "Merck and its allies ganged up on the French.")[21] Perkins's views were quite important since the chief of biologics "controls the discussion . . . gets written comments and decides what to do."[22]

The Biological Standard that WHO adopted created a great deal of outrage. The national honor of both the Netherlands and France were injured, and a new obstacle was created for those interested in a cheap vaccine, especially one produced in the Third World.[23] As far as Prince was concerned, the process that produced the Standard clearly demonstrated the significant level of conflict of interest that permeated the vaccine field. While he was angered at the proceedings, he saw no easy way out of the situation:

> The only guard for decency in these murky situations is in the scientific character [of the individuals]. We all get paid for meetings by manufacturers [and] consult with them. We then sit on advisory committees that affect the future of the companies. Many of us are sensitive to this. . . . The editor of the *New England Journal of Medicine* favors more strict definitions of conflict of interest, disclosure of interest and dealings etc. . . . I would hate to think I would be biased by . . . [company] support—but [unfortunately] some are.[24]

Prince believed, but had no proof, that key supporters of the vaccine standard were acting more as representatives of a specific drug firm than as impartial experts. Unfortunately, he was also perceived by others as similarly compromised. We have already seen that his relationship with Cheil dogged him and the Task Force for years. These mutual recriminations made the fight against undue manufacturer influence extremely difficult.

Maynard and Gust were active for years in lobbying for reopening the vaccine standards question. Both Maynard and Gust wanted people who were closely identified with a particular drug company to be excluded from the deliberations. According to Gust, they found John Petricianni, M.D., acting Chief of Biologicals, sympathetic to their view. (Gust, Maynard, and Petricianni, of the U.S. Food and Drug Administration, were civil servants and forbidden to have close links with pharmaceutical companies.)[25] Petricianni called a new meeting. According to Gust the new session involved "experts not aligned with the manufacturers,"[26] and the resulting new rules were considerably less restrictive. (It is perhaps more accurate to say that the new meeting was dominated not by scientists aligned with Merck, but rather by people close to Pasteur, the Dutch Red Cross, and Cheil.[27] If impartiality did not rule the day, at least competition did, which was a not unhealthy situation.)

The May 1987 Expert Committee on Biologicals meeting in London was very supportive of attempts to legitimize the many different processes employed in vaccine manufacture. It stated[28] that "there are now over 11 licensed manufacturers of plasma-derived hepatitis B vaccines globally. . . . [R]egardless of procedures utilized, these vaccines have been shown to be highly immunogenic and efficacious." The committee went on to suggest that the standards for purity be changed, "that arbitrary specifications of degree of purity [were] no longer appropriate," and "that arbitrary specifications of the nature or number of [inactivation] procedures to be utilized [were] no longer required."

The Paper-Thin Line Between the Task Force and WHO

In November 1987 another important TAG, the Third Meeting of the WHO TAG on Viral Hepatitis, met in Geneva. This meeting produced a report that closely paralleled the Task Force's position on what WHO's hepatitis B policy should look like. Dr. E. A. Ayoola of Nigeria, the Task Force member from Africa, was Vice-Chairman of the meeting, and Maynard, Gust, and Beasley were also present. The Task Force's goal was that the TAG endorse the integration of hepatitis B vaccination into the EPI and lend support to its other goals as well. The report issued by the meeting more than fulfilled those objectives.

The report[29] stated that the recombinant DNA vaccines were not safer or more efficient than plasma and that "plasma-derived vaccines will continue to play an essential role in HB [hepatitis B] control programmes worldwide for the foreseeable future." In addition, it stated that "the dramatic decrease in the price of HB vaccines" now made large-scale vaccination programs feasible and WHO should support them:

The TAG encourages the establishment of programmes and liaising with relevant groups within and without the [World Health] Organization and encourages continued and increasing close collaboration between WHO and such bodies in the development and implementation of the global programme on HB control. . . . The TAG emphatically reiterates that the most important means to control HB on a global scale and to reduce mortality due to chronic sequelae of this infection, including cirrhosis and HCC [hepatocellular carcinoma], is the large scale immunization of infants. It therefore recommends that HB vaccination be integrated into the EPI programme as soon as possible. . . . The first dose . . . should be given as soon as possible after birth. . . . [It] should aim at administration of [the shot] . . . within the first week of life.

These recommendations essentially constituted an endorsement of the Task Force agenda.

The meeting also acknowledged existing weaknesses within WHO that handicapped the fight against hepatitis B. The report said that "a carefully planned and innovative programme for the control of viral hepatitis . . . requires a functioning infrastructure, [and] adequate funding. . . . [Unfortunately,] the viral diseases component of WHO [other than for AIDS] is currently too small to provide the personnel or financial support necessary for a viable programme." It went on to support the WHO viral hepatitis program and "express concern that the funds which had been provided to establish the programme were exhausted." The Task Force wanted WHO involvement increased, and a recognition of the organization's weakness tended to legitimize the Task Force's own activities.

The TAG report clearly demonstrated the importance of Task Force activity at the meeting. However, because this was a high-level WHO meeting, not a Task Force function, its recommendations carried a great deal of objective authority. When dealing with governments and international groups the Task Force could quote the TAG as a source of independent verification of its goals. The unofficial linkage between the two organizations thus operated very effectively in this situation.

Even more important than the November 1987 Hepatitis B TAG report was the position adopted by the EPI Global Advisory Group (GAG) meeting in Washington in the same month. The GAG report recommended that hepatitis B vaccine be integrated into the EPI in countries where the carrier rate was above 2 percent.[30] The Task Force believed that the GAG endorsement constituted the turning point in the hepatitis B struggle because it had made hepatitis B vaccination an official part of the EPI. Unfortunately, the WHO bureaucracy did not interpret this as constituting the organization's formal adoption of the vaccine. (According to Prince, WHO could not act without the cooperation of the United Nations Children's Fund (UNICEF), since it was responsible for finding funding for the EPI vaccines, and UNICEF would not support universal hepatitis B vaccination at that time.)[31]

If the November 1987 meetings were not quite the watershed the Task Force hoped for, they nevertheless had many beneficial results, not the least of which was the fact that the Task Force was made a WHO Collaborating Centre, a unique status for a non-governmental, non-university group. According to Maynard the new status came directly out of conversations he held with two high-ranking WHO officials, Dr. Giorgio Torrigiani (Director, Division of Communicable Diseases) and Dr. Paul Lambert (Chief, Microbiology and Immunology Support Services), after the TAG meeting. Torrigiani wanted the Task Force more closely involved in WHO efforts and saw bestowing the status of Collaborating Centre as the means to insure closer coordination. Maynard, who had headed the Hepatitis B Collaborating Centre while at the Centers for Disease Control (CDC), was exceptionally pleased.

Torrigiani also believed it was necessary for WHO to recruit a full-time staffer to handle its hepatitis B projects. The lack of such a person clearly restricted WHO's ability to be active in that area. The person ultimately chosen for the job was Mark Kane, M.D., of the CDC, who had been instrumental in writing the Thai model project protocol and in preparing the original proposal to the McDonnell Foundation, which had launched the group in the first place.[32] These increasingly power-ful links between the Task Force and WHO, however, did not mean that friction between the two organizations had disappeared—far from it.

A Change in Leadership at WHO Unexpectedly Increases Conflict Between the Task Force and Geneva

In 1988 Dr. Nakajima Hiroshi became Director General of WHO-Geneva. To Maynard and Gust the ascendancy of Nakajima, the man they had worked with in the WPRO Task Force, was a major positive development. They now had someone at the helm who understood and cared about the hepatitis B problem. In keeping with his interest in the issue, Nakajima instructed Torrigiani to draw up a plan for hepa-titis control, with WHO playing a major role and obtaining its own funding. According to Maynard, "this was to be expected, since Dr. Nakajima takes a personal interest in hepatitis B. . . . [However,] while we can all take pride in the fact that our efforts have catalyzed a renewed interest on the part of WHO headquarters, we must be very careful that we are not considered as rivals."[33] This was easier said than done, as Nakajima had demonstrated in China. One of the immediate effects of the new policy was that when a high-ranking WHO official went to Gabon in Africa to establish a model program, the Task Force was not informed beforehand, and Maynard suspected "that this was done so that WHO could demonstrate its independence and its new-found desire to lead rather than [to] follow."[34] There was certainly abundant evidence that not all of Geneva's feelings toward the Task Force were positive.

There was also friction with the leaders of WHO's EPI, the group most concerned with large-scale vaccination in the developing world. Richard Mahoney was told by a knowledgeable source that there were emerging problems for the Task Force in Africa:

He [the informant] said that EPI officials were always being approached by groups who wanted to wipe out this or that disease. He said EPI was having lots of difficulties with the current six vaccines, and it was not helpful to add on more problems. He did not say "you should not burden EPI," but he might as well have. . . . [Key WHO bureaucrats] feel Nakajima will not be supportive of WHO working with the Task Force. . . . They feel that they have a clear green light to proceed on their own. . . . The EPI group may feel we have been too successful and are generating more activity in hepatitis B than they care for. The "burdening EPI" theory will be used as a missile to attack us. We should do what we can to defuse this theory.[35]

Maynard's response was a calm one, because he felt that the normal competitive feelings of WHO leaders could be defused if Task Force members went out of their way to meet with them. As he put it, "In the long run . . . WHO will come to rely on us. They will not, in my opinion, cut off their noses to spite their faces."[36] It is quite clear that despite Mahoney's considerable diplomatic skills, the personal ties to WHO of Maynard and Gust were what was required to harmonize the two organizations. The potential for conflict and disaster was always present.

The Situation in the Philippines

The precariousness of cooperation was well illustrated by the situation that developed in the Philippines. The Task Force had long been interested in working in that country (PATH already had many interests there), but no full-scale model program had been developed. The Task Force decided that in addition to establishing full-scale model programs, it could use the experience it had gained in places such as Thailand and Indonesia to offer its services in an advisory capacity to governments interested in establishing their own national immunization programs. The first opportunity to do this occurred in the Philippines.[37] The Task Force had submitted a proposal to an Australian aid organization for funds to provide technical assistance to the Philippines, but it was declined. Nevertheless, the Philippine Department of Health, which still desired Task Force assistance, had obtained money from the U.S. Agency for International Development-Manila for an expert team to advise it on the establishment of a national hepatitis B program. The advisory group took the form of a collaborative mission between REACH (the Resources for Child Health Project) and PATH (as subcontractor for REACH). Maynard served as the Team Leader, representing PATH and the Task Force simultaneously.[38] The report issued was a far-reaching overview of the situation in the Philippines. Among its observations was that the WPRO-sponsored plasma-for-vaccine exchange program that existed between Manila and the Kitasato Institute of Japan could not meet the requirements of a national vaccine program, and that,

because of the current contentious nature of the competition . . . between the companies which produce hepatitis B vaccines, particularly in respect to unwarranted claims and counter-claims regarding safety and efficacy, it would be wise for the DOH [Department of Health] to avail themselves of the assistance of an unbiased group of international experts in the field . . . such as the International Task Force on Hepatitis B Immunization, in the tender and bid process.[39]

Thus the report amounted, at least in part, to Maynard (i.e., the REACH team) recommending Maynard (the Task Force and PATH) to the Philippine Department of Health, which was exactly what the government wanted. The report's critique of the WPRO's Kitasato Institute plasma-exchange system was the culmination of a Task Force-WHO turf fight begun the year before.

The Philippine Department of Health officials had decided that, starting in 1990, they would include hepatitis B in their EPI, and they wanted Task Force advice. The Task Force was willing to further that goal but was worried about WPRO's attitude:

WPRO sees itself as having undertaken the "missionary" effort in promoting hepatitis B vaccination in the Pacific and has always considered itself as being the leader in these efforts. Also the exchange of plasma to Japan for finishing into vaccine has been a WHO lead effort of which WPRO is quite proud, but it is also very sensitive to the mounting criticism that the process is uneconomical and unsustainable. Despite these criticisms, WPRO clings tenaciously to this mechanism, perhaps as a result of peculiarities of the Japanese mentality regarding "face."[40]

Originally Maynard believed that it was important not to initiate any action without WHO approval. However, with the Philippine's Secretary of Health planning to send the Task Force a formal invitation to help, he felt it would be virtually impossible for WHO to refuse to cooperate.[41]

Nevertheless, when the issue actually arose, "WPRO was unwilling to agree to a cooperative effort with the Task Force.... [Rather,] WHO... informed the DOH [Department of Health] that the Task Force ... [was] 'duplicating the efforts of WHO.' "[42] WPRO proposed to offer the Philippine government either technology transfer or participation in the plasma-exchange program, both of which would involve the Kitasato Institute of Japan.[43] (The key figure in these heated negotiations was Dr. Umenai Takusai, who later followed Nakajima to Geneva as his trusted advisor.) The Task Force wanted to calm relations with WPRO—but not at the expense of failing to aid the Philippine government. By the time of the REACH report, it was determined to go forward with or without WPRO's blessing.

Alternating conflict and cooperation between WHO and the Task Force has been a continuing theme in their relationship, as has been the need for skillful diplomacy. The issues between the two groups have often been of fundamental importance.

The Task Force Versus the Major Pharmaceutical Companies and Their Scientific Supporters

One of the chief repercussions of the important 1987 TAG meeting was that Torrigiani of WHO decided that the TAG had served its purpose and a smaller steering committee was needed to provide guidance for future activities concerning hepatitis B. In keeping with that belief (and consistent with the TAG's own recommendation), a committee headed by Friedrich Deinhardt, M.D., an internationally respected German hepatitis expert, was established. Over the years there had been constant conflict between Task Force members and Deinhardt. Deinhardt had been active in setting up the original WHO Biological Standard for hepatitis B vaccines and had opposed all attempts to liberalize these requirements. Task Force members constantly questioned his objectivity because in their eyes he was too closely associated with Merck to maintain credibility.[44] According to Maynard, once the standards were relaxed, Deinhardt heavily lobbied to get the old standards reestablished. Maynard felt that Deinhardt's goal was to use the committee for attacks on the Cheil and KGCC vaccines, both of which he strongly opposed.

As Chairperson of the TAG, Deinhardt wanted to set up a formal review committee to approve all model hepatitis B project proposals— those directly under WHO auspices and those of WHO Collaborating Centres. This goal seemed aimed directly at the Task Force. Maynard's response was to make clear that acceptance of Collaborating Centre status did not mean the Task Force was willing to have its independent actions supervised or controlled by WHO. That kind of honor it did not need, and Maynard had the prestige to make his position stick.[45]

SmithKline Initiates a Second Generation of Vaccine Wars

Deinhardt also played a significant role in one of the most important and threatening challenges to be directed at the Task Force: an attempt to impugn the safety and efficacy of the Cheil and KGCC vaccines. The attack came from one of the largest pharmaceutical houses, SmithKline.

The most important drug companies had been engaged in murderous attacks on each other ever since the hepatitis B vaccine had come on the market. In Europe, Pasteur and Merck, the original manufacturers, had played upon the public's fear of AIDS to discredit each other's products. The disastrous result was the reluctance of individuals at high risk of hepatitis B virus infection to use either of the new vaccines.

This type of commercial warfare was continued outside of Europe and was adopted by other companies as they developed their own variants of the vaccine. When SmithKline entered the hepatitis B field by producing a recombinant DNA vaccine, a number of Task Force members reacted very favorably. SmithKline, in contrast to the other companies, seemed to reject the idea that hepatitis B treatment should be a boutique vaccine geared primarily to the middle classes. Rather, it set its sights on the potentially limitless mass market, a development that was consistent with the Task Force's own goals.[46] Unfortunately, there was a down side to this broader vision. Insofar as SmithKline was out for large markets, it became exceptionally aggressive in its relationships with competitors. Most ominously, since it only made a recombinant DNA vaccine, it started to attack plasma-derived vaccines as dangerous to the public's health. (Merck, which also produced a recombinant DNA vaccine, did not adopt such a policy. It is perhaps not irrelevant to note that Merck continued to manufacture its original plasma vaccine.)[47] One of the first places SmithKline used this destructive marketing approach was in New Zealand.

SmithKline in New Zealand

Alexander Milne, a hospital-based laboratory technician, had inadvertently discovered in the early 1980s that New Zealand suffered from a hepatitis B problem similar to that of the developing world. The Maori population had carrier rates that matched those of other Pacific Islanders and mainland Asians. Most of the transmission of the disease occurred horizontally, from child to child, and much of it took place in elementary schools. In areas having a high proportion of Maoris in the population, infection of children was widespread. Milne, lacking medical credentials, found it exceptionally hard to convince public health officials of the extent of the danger. Nevertheless, he dedicated himself to alerting the population to the problem and pushed for universal childhood immunization. He functioned as a one-man task force, and to support his fight he brought in hepatitis experts from abroad— including Maynard, Gust, and Prince—to strengthen his case.

After Milne succeeded in persuading the government of the seriousness of the problem, New Zealand proceeded to purchase Merck plasma vaccine for a mass immunization program, whereupon Smith-Kline entered the scene. As Maynard put it in a letter to the head of the Pan-American Health Organization (PAHO), "I have seen an excellent national hepatitis B immunization program in New Zealand placed in extreme jeopardy by the unwarranted fights between rival manufacturers."[48] The problem was that SmithKline tried to exploit existing fears in the population:

As one might expect there is always a conservative anti-vaccination group in most developed countries that will make the most of any subliminal fears that might exist in the general population about the safety of any pharmaceutical or biological product.[49]

The company circulated a marketing brochure that raised the specter of plasma vaccine disease transmission, and thereby created a crisis in public confidence.[50] Nevertheless, the New Zealand program survived.

SmithKline Attacks the Task Force in the Caribbean

SmithKline's next attack was aimed at the Task Force, and specifically the Cheil and KGCC vaccines that it utilized. The assault came in the form of an anonymous document leaked to the PAHO. (PAHO represented WHO in the Americas.) The material was a frontal attack on Cheil that impugned the Task Force and especially its Chairman, Alfred Prince.[51]

The document was sent by PAHO to WHO in Geneva, where it was distributed. Deinhardt, both as a member of the Hepatitis B TAG and as the head of a WHO Collaborating Centre, received a copy.[52] Relatively quickly the material was identified as a SmithKline internal marketing memo designed to help salesmen influence customers. The memo highlighted perceived weaknesses in the Cheil Sugar Company and its vaccine that could be exploited. For example, it pointed out that Cheil used a heat-deactivation method that the Dutch Red Cross had pioneered but that the Dutch had withdrawn its vaccine from the market because of problems. It also claimed that Cheil promoted its product as originating from its Genetic Engineering Division, an assertion that "was presumably [designed] to mislead customers into thinking it is genetically engineered."[53] The memo advised salesmen to "make sure the customers are aware of this and discredit Cheil Sugar for using misleading promotion; how can any information be trusted, how else might they be trying to fool the customer?"[54] It went on to raise questions about Cheil's dosage, safety, testing, immunogenicity, and protective efficacy. It concluded:

Public health officials have been demanding a reduction in the price of hepatitis B vaccines. . . . Cheil Sugar has replied to this demand by producing a cheap vaccine. However, in order to arrive at the reduction in price, quality and safety have had to be traded. The vaccinee and very often physicians are unaware of this and someone presumed protected may in fact be at immediate risk.[55]

The memo also contained an attack on the Task Force's objectivity, based on the fact that Prince was involved in developing the Cheil vaccine.

Before the source of the memo was ascertained, the PAHO took the document quite seriously because PAHO was officially sponsoring a field trial utilizing the Cheil vaccine on the island of St. Kitts. The document also seemed to reflect badly on the ethics of WHO.[56]

Maynard made it clear to Francisco Pinheiro, head of PAHO, that the circulation of "anonymous or company-specific marketing documents"[57] was inappropriate for WHO. Pinheiro agreed and said he would ask Geneva to stop circulating the memo until its origins could be ascertained. A few days later Maynard informed Pinheiro that Task Force members attending a meeting with SmithKline in Belgium were told that the document was indeed an internal paper of that company. As such, Maynard maintained, it had no scientific standing and was not worthy of WHO consideration.

Notwithstanding that fact, the document continued to exert significant negative influence. It provided Deinhardt ammunition to attack Cheil, undermine the Task Force, and reiterate his hostility to the liberalized Biological Standard.[58] Deinhardt accepted the legitimacy of all of the points raised in the SmithKline document and rejected out of hand the reply Cheil had prepared. He summarized his own position by saying, "I cannot endorse the use of . . . [the Cheil vaccine] in any vaccination projects in which WHO is directly or indirectly [i.e., as in Task Force Model Programs] involved until the questions raised are answered satisfactorily."[59] He went on to strongly advise against beginning the St. Kitts hepatitis B trials using the Cheil vaccine.[60] Maynard believed "that Deinhardt is . . . trying to completely reopen the work of the WHO Expert Committee on Biologicals, by forcing the convening of a small external committee,"[61] and while he did not know how WHO would respond, he saw the danger as very real.

(It is important to realize that although Task Force members were suspicious of Deinhardt's motivation, there were in fact good reasons for Deinhardt to be skeptical of the Cheil vaccine. As we have seen earlier, Prince and Maynard constantly had to badger Cheil to carry out proper trials for the vaccine and to conduct itself in a manner that met international scientific standards. The Koreans were more competent in mastering the substance of vaccine manufacturing than the appearance of such proficiency. The fact that Deinhardt was suspicious and unwilling to give Cheil the benefit of the doubt did not require the existence of ulterior motives on his part. However, given an international system in which scientists are economically linked to commercial companies, and given that the concept of conflict of interest is not well defined, suspicions of unethical motivation are both inevitable and ubiquitous. They severely poison the collegial atmosphere among scientists.)

To counteract Deinhardt's damaging actions, Maynard wrote him a letter[62] in which he made a point-by-point critique of the SmithKline document's factual assertions and also provided a defense of the St. Kitts project—a program that had been originally planned at the CDC when he was Chief of the Hepatitis Branch. At the same time, without directly accusing Deinhardt, Maynard pointed out that "scurrilous comments"—to the effect that the Task Force, its Chairman, Alfred Prince, and Cheil had an unacceptable (i.e., commercial) relationship—had been overheard at the last WHO Scientific Advisory Group of Experts (SAGE) meeting in Geneva. Maynard insisted that such remarks needed to be avoided because they led to unfounded rumors. (As an example of how dangerous high-level hostility could be, Maynard had learned that Dr. Natth of Thailand had become so upset by "a senior member of the SAGE's" claim that the Task Force and Prince were "in bed with Cheil" that he contemplated suggesting that the opening ceremony of the Thai project be canceled.)[63]

In addition to the anti-Cheil material, the Task Force got hold of a SmithKline document being circulated in Saudi Arabia that just as aggressively attacked the credibility of the KGCC vaccine.[64] Maynard sent the material to KGCC, noting,

You should be aware that the history of marketing competition in the Western world regarding hepatitis B vaccine has been one of attack and counterattack by the companies who have manufactured the vaccine. This form of behavior is not new. [However,] our Task Force, as an international group of scientists and public health experts, as well as a WHO Collaborating Centre, cannot become involved in these competitive interactions between manufacturers.[65]

Maynard also informed Cheil that for the Task Force to be seen as "involved on the side of one or another company [in such litigious interactions] could do grievous harm to our mission."[66] Thus he demanded that the Task Force be consulted and notified before any documents with legal implications were sent out with its name.

It is important to recognize that while the commercially inspired attacks on KGCC and Cheil were basically unfair, they were not totally groundless, which makes it less unreasonable that someone like Deinhardt would be persuaded by them. Both companies clearly tried to misdirect purchasers about important aspects of their product. For example, in a document prepared for KGCC to present to the government of Kenya, there was an attempt to hide the Korean origin of the vaccine and give the impression that it was made in Britain. The work also implied that the vaccine was WHO-approved, when WHO does not actually approve any vaccine but rather establishes requirements that vaccines may or may not meet. It was also true that Cheil in some of its material did speak of its vaccine as coming out of its genetic engineering laboratory, creating the false impression that it was a recombinant DNA vaccine.

The Task Force Wins Over SmithKline

While the Task Force avoided any legal involvement in the dispute, it nevertheless did everything it could informally to end the attacks. In keeping with this goal a meeting was arranged with the heads of SmithKline in Belgium. Typically, the Task Force attempted to avoid a direct confrontation with SmithKline so as to create an opportunity for future cooperation between the two organizations. In its characteristic way, the Task Force sought not simply to prevent hostile attacks but to forge links that would turn erstwhile enemies into allies. This was especially true in the case of SmithKline, because the company's aggressiveness came out of its desire to create a mass hepatitis B vaccine market, which was already a progressive and pioneering attitude for a large pharmaceutical house.

A good example of positive results issuing out of highly irresponsible commercial aggressiveness occurred in the Philippines. In that country, SmithKline started an educational campaign that was quite inflammatory. According to an outraged Dr. Mario Taguiwalo, the Philippine Undersecretary of Health and Chief of Staff, SmithKline "is a company whose marketing of Hepatitis B vaccine is increasingly descending to the bottom of the ethical barrel . . . [by] creat[ing] unjustified widespread fear . . . among low-risk [adult] groups"[67] while it aggressively offered discount group hepatitis B vaccination and lobbied to make hepatitis B immunization a legal requirement. The Task Force was opposed to such panic-creating recklessness, but it could not ignore the fact that these tactics generated a lot of political pressure to make the government get serious about hepatitis B.

To resolve the conflict, a high-level meeting of the SmithKline leadership and the Task Force was arranged. Mahoney told SmithKline point-blank that attacks on the safety of plasma vaccines constituted attacks on the Task Force. If SmithKline persisted, the Task Force would be forced to fight the company and to do so publicly. SmithKline responded that the company's strategy was simply based upon market research showing that individuals were not being immunized with plasma-derived vaccine because of fears regarding its safety, and Smith-Kline wanted it known that its recombinant DNA vaccine did not have any such associations. Nevertheless, the SmithKline leadership promised not to demean the safety of the plasma vaccines in the future. The Task Force members also insisted that the attacks on Cheil must cease. The SmithKline official said they were shocked that the internal memos had been made public and denied they had given approval for it.[68] After the two groups reviewed the whole series of areas where they had conflicted and discussed how they might resolve them, talk began about the possibility of future large-scale cooperation.[69]

The two groups spoke about the possibility that SmithKline would make a sizable contribution to a model program in Africa. The company made it clear that it did not want to contribute to a project in a country that was sufficiently prosperous that it might be able to purchase vaccine in the near future. The Task Force countered that it was not worth its while to work in a country so poor that it could not pay for a long-term program after the demonstration project ended, or in one whose EPI was too underdeveloped. They agreed that Kenya seemed to meet both groups' requirements.[70]

SmithKline outlined its pricing policy for the vaccine: The company would always price its product above the Korean vaccines in order to maintain its image. Mahoney countered that the Task Force would not back down from its own commitment to $1 a dose, but that the two positions could be reconciled if SmithKline donated an amount of vaccine to the model program so that the total (donated and purchased) average price was $1 a shot. The Task Force was nothing if not flexible in pursuit of its goals.

At a later meeting, Maynard told SmithKline officials that there existed "a suspicion on our part that SKB [SmithKline Biologicals] was actively trying to exclude the Task Force from participation in important international meetings that were supported in part by SKB."[71] SmithKline strongly denied this, and Maynard accepted the denials as sincere. With that issue out of the way, they discussed the company's desire to donate 100,000 doses of vaccine to a Task Force program in Africa and their intention that the donated and purchased price would in fact equal $1 a dose. When asked if Kenya would be acceptable as the project country, the company leaders said "we have a deal"[72]—and thus began a new phase in their relationship. Maynard believed the turnabout was at least partially due to the Task Force's newly acquired status as a WHO Collaborating Centre, which impressed SmithKline and forced them to realize "that we are a potent force that must be dealt with differently from the way they would deal with a rival company."[73] All in all, Task Force diplomacy and skill changed a crisis into an opportunity to advance the fight against hepatitis B.

The Task Force's skills in turning a problem into an advantage is nowhere better illustrated than in the group's response to the Smith-Kline offer of donated vaccine. Up to that point the Task Force had shied away from accepting free vaccine for its projects for fear that the donor would get a public relations bonanza, but the long-term effect would not be a lower price. Instead, the Task Force preferred the bid and tender approach developed during the Indonesian project. However, after the SmithKline offer, the Task Force decided it would indeed accept donated vaccine, but only if the company met three conditions:

The company will agree that [a] single dose of hepatitis B vaccine, when procured by the public sector in large scale, will cost no more than $1/dose . . . The company will agree that it is seriously considering the development of a multivalent vaccine of DPT-HBV [diphtheria-pertussis-tetanus/hepatitis B virus], and agrees that, in large scale sales to the public sector, the HBV component will cost no more than $.50/dose.[74]

Those were very stiff terms to demand of a company planning to donate 100,000 doses of vaccine, but the Task Force succeeded in getting SmithKline to meet them.[75]

Ultimately, the Task Force found it could work successfully not only with SmithKline but with other large pharmaceutical houses as well. Merck, which had for years ignored the possibility of mass market hepatitis B programs, had a major change of heart and became interested.[76] The end of the boutique vaccine mentality meant that competition and lower prices became the norm in the hepatitis B area. This was exactly what the Task Force had hoped for, and the developing world reaped the benefits.[77]

* * *

In summary, whether dealing with WHO or pharmaceutical companies, the Task Force membership always put the goal of fighting hepatitis B above the pleasures of self-righteousness, ego, or revenge. They did not shy away from battle or competition, but neither did they work to destroy or humiliate their opponents. Rather, they worked to solve the problem at hand and then convert their enemies into allies. This was not easily done—either emotionally or practically—but they persisted. Pursuing that policy was largely responsible for their ultimate success.

The Task Force's ability to maintain such a reconciliatory position appears little less than miraculous, given the degree of conflict that existed on the international level. Whether the stage was China, the Philippines, the Caribbean, or Geneva, good and sufficient reasons always existed for disagreement rather than cooperation. Of course, it takes two to make an agreement, and ultimately both WHO and the large drug companies had to be willing to compromise. This goal was made possible by the Task Force's willingness to take the first step.

Notes

1. Interview with James Maynard, June 18, 1991.
2. For some of the rivalry between WHO and the EPI, see Jack W. Hopkins, *The Eradication of Smallpox: Organizational Learning and Innovation in International Health* (Boulder, Colo.: Westview Press, 1989), 40–67.
3. Interview with Maynard, June 18, 1991.
4. Interview with Warren, Director of Health Science for the Maxwell/Macmillan Foundation, November 18, 1991. Also see Jack W. Hopkins, *The Eradication of Smallpox,* 51–52, 83–84, for observations supportive of this view.
5. Interview with James Maynard, June 18, 1991.
6. Ibid.
7. Ibid.
8. Ibid.
9. Letter from Richard Mahoney to Dr. John Bruer, President of the McDonnell Foundation, April 20, 1987.
10. Ibid.
11. Ibid.
12. "Report to the Minister of Public Health, Professor Chen Minzhang, People's Republic of China, on PRODUCTION AND DISTRIBUTION OF HEPATITIS B VACCINE," submitted by the International Task Force on Hepatitis B Immunization and PATH, September 1987.
13. Dr. Xu Xi-Yi was also a consultant, and he was the Task Force member from China.
14. "Hepatitis B Immunization Program in Long An County, China," Second Technical and Financial Report to the International Development Research Centre by Guangxi Anti-Epidemic Station and PATH (Canada), October 1990. While the Task Force was very excited by the apparent capability for hepatitis B vaccine storage at room temperatures, they had to be very careful not to publicize that possibility prematurely. Dr. Violet How (and Dr. Mark Kane, who was visiting the Task Force) was very concerned that nothing be done until the findings were clearly confirmed, for fear of confusing local authorities (Task Force meeting in Houston, 1990).
15. "Report of the Third Meeting of the WHO Technical Advisory Group on Viral Hepatitis," WHO, Geneva, November 2–5, 1987, 13.
16. Interview with Alfred Prince, March 27, 1991.
17. See *World Health Organization Technical Report Series, 658: WHO Expert Committee on Biological Standardization, Thirty-first Report* (Geneva: WHO, 1981).
18. In reply to a letter from the Director of the Malaysian National Blood Transfusion Service, Maynard spelled out the role of WHO biological requirements for hepatitis B vaccines: "WHO, as an international agency of the United Nations[,] does not act as a licensing authority. In this regard, it is unlike national licensing authorities which give approval to the distribution and marketing of biological products within their jurisdictions. WHO does not issue 'approvals,' nor does it regulate the transfer or distribution of these products in international markets. On the other hand, WHO, through its Expert Committee on Biologicals, does formulate 'Biological Requirements' for certain" products (letter by Maynard, to Dr. G. Duraisamy, May 6, 1988). The problem was that many nations saw a failure to meet WHO requirements as proof of a dangerous product.

19. All quotes are from an interview with Prince, January 22, 1991.

20. Prince's unhappiness about the way biologic standards were set was shared, interestingly enough, by officials at Merck—though not necessarily in this particular case. In a conference held in 1992, Merck officials commented that "WHO specifications for vaccines . . . are established by Expert Committees and initially may include representatives of companies which manufacture the vaccines in addition to WHO administrative staff as well as outside scientific experts. This does not guarantee that specifications will have been derived from well-established scientific tests but may include some arbitrary decisions based partially on fact and extrapolated logic" (Kenneth R. Brown and R. Gordon Douglas Jr. [President of Merck Vaccine Division], "New Challenges in Quality Control and Licensure: Regulation," 5, draft of a paper presented at the Conference on Vaccines and Public Health, Bethesda, Maryland, November 5–6, 1992, sponsored by the National Institute on Allergy and Infectious Diseases).

21. Interview with Gust, February 24, 1991.

22. Interview with Prince, January 22, 1991.

23. Letter from Prince to John Petricianni, Chief, Biologics, WHO, February 18, 1987.

24. Interview with Prince, January 22, 1991.

25. While they were allowed to participate in field studies, they could not consult for personal profit.

26. Interview with Gust, February 24, 1991.

27. Ibid. His testimony is a bit contradictory here.

28. The modified WHO standards were repeated and highlighted in "Report: Working Group on Hepatitis B," convened by the WPRO, Seoul, South Korea, August 1987, published March 1988, 2–3. Task Force members Maynard, Beasley, and Gust were present at this meeting. The report has a Task Force tone to it; the Task Force was active in both the London and Seoul meetings.

29. "Report of the Third Meeting of the WHO Technical Advisory Group on Viral Hepatitis," WHO, Geneva, November 2–3, 1987 (unpublished).

30. "Report of the Expanded Programme on Immunization Global Advisory Group Meeting," held November 9–13, 1987, Washington, D.C. (WHO: Geneva, 1987), which said, "Countries with chronic carrier rates of hepatitis B of over 2% and with the resources to initiate hepatitis B immunization programmes should introduce hepatitis B immunization as an integral part of existing childhood immunization programs." Beasley was an observer at the meeting.

31. Interview with Prince, March 27, 1991. Prince believes that UNICEF's head, James Grant, "shot it down." In a memo from Richard Mahoney to Maynard dated June 20, 1988, he talks about a UNICEF meeting on June 16, 1988, at which Dr. V. Ramalingaswami, Special Advisor to the Executive Director of UNICEF, "also seems to support the view that hepatitis B, despite the GAG decisions of November 1987, is not yet an 'official' part of EPI."

32. Interview with Kane, May 5, 1992. He went to St. Louis with the Task Force founding group to make the original presentation to the McDonnell Foundation and helped write the Thai protocol, both in the capacity as a CDC aide to Maynard. The appointment of Kane represented a marked increase in WHO's support and interest in hepatitis B. He was placed as the head of the hepatitis subunit within Microbiology and Immunology Support Services.

33. Memo by Maynard to Task Force members, July 8, 1988.

34. Ibid.

35. Memo by Mahoney to Maynard, July 12, 1988.

36. Memo by Maynard to Hepatitis B File, July 25, 1988.

37. "1990 Annual Narrative and Financial Report to the James S. McDonnell Foundation from the International Task Force on Hepatitis B Immunization," March 1991. The report says the decision was made at the 1990 meeting of the Task Force, but clearly the policy was in effect in the Philippines long before that meeting.

38. See "The Integration of Hepatitis B Immunization into EPI in the Philippines," September 1990, The REACH Project.

39. Ibid.

40. Memo by Maynard to Leona D'Agnes, October 16, 1989.

41. Ibid.

42. Memo by Mahoney to Maynard, May 11, 1990.

43. Ibid.

44. I tried to contact Dr. Deinhardt to set up an interview to hear his side of the story, but I discovered he had died a week before I sent my fax.

45. Memo by Maynard to Task Force members, January 24, 1989.

46. Interview with Gust, February 24, 1991. Prince has been very vocal in his belief that SmithKline was different from other drug companies and has been an asset in the fight against hepatitis B (interview with Prince, September 12, 1990). Maynard also has seen them as separate from other drug companies (interview with Maynard, June 1991).

47. Interview with Maynard, June 19, 1991.

48. Letter from Maynard to Dr. Francisco Pinheiro of PAHO, July 20, 1988.

49. Memo by Maynard to Task Force members, June 11, 1988.

50. Ibid. SmithKline's position on the safety of the plasma-based hepatitis B vaccine was not its only action to create a negative effect in that part of the world. The Australian Pharmaceutical Manufacturers' Association (APMA) felt that SmithKline had violated its code of conduct when the company targeted schools in a promotional campaign that suggested that all pupils should be vaccinated with their vaccine. The APMA felt that the campaign gave unbalanced information and was directly aimed at the public—a violation of its rules. Rather than comply with the APMA's code, SmithKline resigned from the organization (Andrew Chetley, *Healthy Business? World Health and the Pharmaceutical Industry* [London: Zed Books Ltd., 1990], 56).

51. Memo by Maynard to Task Force members, June 11, 1988.

52. Memo by Mahoney to Maynard, July 12, 1988; memo by Maynard to Task Force members, July 8, 1988.

53. Anonymous document, (PAHO/WHO stamped on top, dated 5/6/88) attached to a letter from Whitman and Ransom (lawyers for Cheil Sugar) to SmithKline Beckman Corporation, dated July 26, 1988.

54. Ibid.

55. Ibid.

56. Memo by Maynard to Mahoney, May 6, 1988, relating a conversation with Francisco Pinheiro of PAHO.

57. Ibid.

58. Letter from Deinhardt to Dr. Yuri Ghendon of WHO, June 7, 1988.

59. Letter from Deinhardt to Dr. Yuri Ghendon of WHO, June 14, 1988.

60. Ibid.

61. Memo by Maynard to Shin Seung-il, July 28, 1988.

62. Memo by Maynard to Deinhardt, August 29, 1988.

63. Memo by Maynard to Gust, August 1, 1988.

64. There was also a major attack on the KGCC vaccine in "Hepatitis B Vaccine Contract Goes to Untested Product," in *Nature,* September 3, 1987; as well as an attack on Cheil in "Cheap Hepatitis B Vaccine Divides Health Experts," in *New Scientist,* June 11, 1987. Both articles utilized material supplied by a SmithKline spokesman. The Task Force was quick to protest distortions in both articles. See the letter from Maynard to the Deputy Editor of *Nature,* September 22, 1987, as an example.

65. Memo by Maynard to Mr. Y. C. Yoo, Managing Director of KGCC, July 18, 1988.

66. Memo by Maynard to Shin Seung-il, July 28, 1988.

67. Editorial, "Hepatitis B Vaccine—A Company Goldmine," in *EPI Newsletter, Expanded Program on Immunization in the Philippines,* July–December 1989.

68. Maynard accepted their claims and said he felt the top managers were honest people but their reasonable approach "did not come across to the marketing level," which functioned as independent decision centers (interview with Maynard, June 19, 1991).

69. Memo by Mahoney to Maynard, May 18, 1988.

70. Ibid. Apparently, SmithKline had thought of working with the Task Force for some time. When it looked like that would not be possible, SmithKline offered UNICEF a contribution of 100,000 doses of vaccine for the first year of a project, and then additional contributions in later years. With cooperation now possible, SmithKline officials did not want to withdraw their offer. The Task Force told them that was no problem and they would like to work with both SmithKline and UNICEF. Later, UNICEF rejected the offer but referred the company to the Task Force as a good alternative (memo by Maynard to Task Force members, July 8, 1988).

71. Memo by Maynard to Hepatitis B File, July 25, 1988.

72. Ibid.

73. Ibid.

74. Memo by Mahoney to Robert Hackett of SmithKline, December 14, 1988.

75. Letter from Mahoney to Dr. Philip Hallwood, SmithKline, March 30, 1989. Maynard put the issue of getting free vaccine in an amusing way: "The Task Force doesn't beg money from drug companies; PATH does. That is where [the Task Force's famous] flexibility comes in." However, to protect themselves from the appearance of being influenced, "we don't favor any one company, we solicit all [of them]." The need to be independent of the taint of conflict of interest vis-à-vis the drug companies was also important as it affected individual Task Force members. Some of the original members of the Task Force had received grants to evaluate different vaccines. The question arose whether Task Force members should repudiate such money. A major debate took place, and the group decided that it was legitimate to accept money provided that no one received personal funds (e.g., it was all right for the University of Texas to receive drug company funds that Beasley administered if he received no direct remuneration). Prince was encouraged to give up his Cheil royalties, which he did (interview with Maynard, June 19, 1991).

76. Maynard said he had for years despaired about Merck's philosophy of marketing, which seemed to be: "We do not want to be in a competitive market,

we want to make our profit in a small, high priced market." He believed that Task Force pressure was at least partially responsible for their change of policy. They started to become interested in the international public sector competition, which benefited the entire developing world (interview with Maynard, June 19, 1991).

77. One result was that SmithKline could alert the Task Force that KGCC was not abiding by its Indonesian agreement to offer the $1-per-dose price to all public authorities and that SmithKline was actually offering the cheapest vaccine on the market. While Task Force members were not convinced that the accusation was totally accurate (because of dose and price differences between adults and children), they appreciated SmithKline's desire to compete on price (letter from Robert Hackett, International Marketing Director, SmithKline, to Mahoney, January 4, 1989; reply from Maynard to Hackett, January 16, 1989).

Chapter 6
On the Road to Victory: Hepatitis B as the Seventh Universal Vaccine

This chapter deals with the expansion of the Task Force's efforts into Africa, the Middle East, and the former Soviet Union. As the Task Force's prestige and influence grew it was called upon by individual governments, multi-national corporations, and the World Health Organization (WHO) to aid in a variety of anti-hepatitis B programs. It set up two full-scale model projects in Africa, but its other interventions were equally important. As in its earlier work the Task Force found that the array of conflicting interests in each country challenged its ability to maintain both its independence and its good reputation.

This chapter also details the Task Force's crowning achievement: the adoption of hepatitis B vaccine as the seventh universal vaccine by the Expanded Programme on Immunization (EPI) of WHO. This was the goal to which all Task Force efforts were aimed from the time of the group's formation. The following will explore the political situation that made this victory possible.

Despite the EPI's official adoption of hepatitis B vaccine, the crucial problem of financing large-scale immunization programs in the developing world still remains. Unfortunately for the Task Force, the key to funding universal hepatitis B vaccination is held by the United Nations Children's Fund (UNICEF), which continues to oppose the new mandate. UNICEF's objections to hepatitis B as the seventh universal vaccine had many facets, and the Task Force had to expend much effort to win UNICEF's cooperation.

This chapter ends with a review of the accomplishments of the Task Force and the lessons its history teaches us about working in the international health arena.

* * *

During the period that the Task Force was intensely focused on the model projects in Indonesia, Thailand, and China, it never forgot that Africa also suffered severely from the hepatitis B pandemic. Task Force members knew, however, that unlike the situation in Asia, no widespread governmental awareness or concern with the problem existed. For most Africans, the continent suffered from so many pressing health problems that hepatitis B simply seemed to lack urgency. Nevertheless, there were 50,000,000 chronic carriers of the disease in Africa, of whom 12,500,000 would ultimately die of liver disease. In countries such as Cameroon, carriership was 10–25 percent of the population and liver cancer was the number one cause of cancer mortality, with hepatitis B accounting for fully 3 percent of total deaths.[1]

The Kenya Model Hepatitis B Project

The Task Force wanted to set up two model projects in Africa: one in an anglophone nation, the other in a francophone nation. It was hoped that the models would serve as exemplars for their linguistic neighbors. For a nation to be a candidate for a model program the country had to be prosperous enough to sustain the program after the project ended, it had to have a functioning EPI, and it had to have the full commitment of the political leadership. The first country that met these conditions was Kenya.

As we have seen in an earlier chapter, WHO officials in Africa opposed a Task Force initiative; they felt that the EPI was already overburdened in most countries and that hepatitis B would completely overwhelm it.[2] When the Task Force assessed the feasibility of working in Kenya, it was keenly aware of the need to convince all parties that adding hepatitis B to the EPI would help rather than hurt that effort. It was especially important in Kenya to convince the U.S. Agency for International Development (USAID) of that fact in order to avoid the agency's active opposition.[3] Richard Mahoney felt that establishing a hepatitis project could significantly reinvigorate the EPI by providing additional training, working to stimulate renewed enthusiasm among vaccinators, and expanding the research effort to discover the obstacles to effective delivery of the six existing EPI vaccines. In addition, the project could help establish a pregnancy and birth registration system that would be helpful to the EPI.[4]

Kenya, like Indonesia, seemed ripe for Task Force intervention in part because of the deadly effects of hepatitis B on prominent individuals. As Mahoney put it, "We were told there was commitment in the ministry to dealing with hepatitis and that this commitment originated, in large part, from several liver cancer deaths among important individuals."[5] As in Indonesia, the Program for Appropriate Technology in Health (PATH) had been active in Kenya, and it wanted to establish a permanent office there.[6]

Many differences existed in the epidemiology of hepatitis B in Africa and Southeast Asia. One of the most important was that in Asia perinatal (i.e, mother to child) transmission was a significant source of infection, a fact that necessitated giving the vaccination as close to birth as possible. In Africa, horizontal (i.e., child to child) transmission between children was the overwhelming means by which the disease spread. This latter situation allowed for a more flexible approach to the timing of vaccination.[7]

The Task Force found the Kenya EPI staff to be well aware of the hepatitis B problem and to be interested in integrating it into their program, but the price of the vaccine, at $1 a dose, was still too high for Kenya. The health staff pointed out, however, that "offering hepatitis B vaccine to themselves and senior political leaders and their families would be a good means to obtain enthusiasm for the program for the leaders, as well as the population at large."[8] The Task Force was not opposed to offering free vaccine to civil administrators, health officials, and their families, but it lacked the money to do so. It was willing, however, to encourage the vaccine manufacturer to donate what was needed.

In the final analysis the Kenya program turned out to be the most politicized and difficult of all the Task Force's model projects. Kenya had a reputation as being a difficult country in which to work for nongovernmental organizations. As James Maynard[9] put it, "Kenyans like to bite the hands that feed them," and unfortunately the country lived up to that reputation. However, the Kenya project offered a major opportunity "to get things moving in Africa" and to convince other African countries of both the severity of the hepatitis problem and the possibility of successfully dealing with it. According to Maynard, "All our projects are aimed at making it almost impossible for a government not to continue with hepatitis B immunization after we quit," and Kenya, its difficulties notwithstanding, had the resources to do just that.

The Cameroon Model Project

The second African model project was established in Cameroon, West Africa—a nation with both anglophone and francophone areas. This project was a joint WHO-Task Force collaboration. The Cameroon program was designed not only to demonstrate the feasibility of a mass hepatitis B vaccination program, but also to investigate the possibility of going beyond the cold chain and the viability of a quadrivalent (four-antigen) diphtheria-pertussis-tetanus-hepatitis B virus vaccine.

The possibility of giving the hepatitis vaccine in a single shot along with three of the established EPI vaccines was exceptionally attractive to the Task Force, which was very supportive of all scientific research that might lessen the need for frequent child–health system contacts. The Task Force wanted not only to combine vaccines but also to reduce the number of hepatitis B shots required—for example, through a time-release injection or some other method. Interestingly enough, the Cameroon project was made possible only because the Task Force was able to convince Merck Sharp and Dohme to provide approximately 248,000 doses of recombinant DNA vaccine to the program.[10]

As in other projects, the Task Force put significant effort into discovering the impediments and constraints that might undermine the new program. A series of supervisory tours, undertaken to check out the efficiency of the general Cameroon EPI, uncovered major shortcomings which, if not corrected, would subvert the program. Especially worrisome was the lack of careful temperature monitoring, the frequent absence of steam sterilizers, and the shortage of needles and syringes (which manifested itself in the re-use of unsterilized needles on different children). Management problems made firm control over vaccination activities and patient follow-up difficult to maintain. All these findings underscored the necessity of maintaining close monitoring and supervision of the program.[11]

In both Kenya and Cameroon the Task Force and PATH continued to be dedicated to providing an educational component within each project. In Kenya the use of field workers was seen as exceptionally important in sensitizing the community to the importance of the hepatitis issue. Local health educators, public health people, and field workers galvanized their communities into enthusiastic cooperation. Special workshops were set up to provide the workers with the technical information they needed.

The fundamental importance of public education and understanding for the success of the projects was driven home in Cameroon by a study supported by PATH and the University of Yaounde.[12] Shortly before the hepatitis B campaign was to begin, an anti-tetanus toxoid program had been initiated in the English-speaking northwestern part of the country. The vaccination of young girls in a part of Cameroon that felt alienated from the government and that was pro-natalist at a time when the government favored restricting the birth rate led to terrifying rumors that the vaccination program was really a secret attempt to sterilize the young women. These rumors were so firmly rooted that the study found it advisable to delay the official opening ceremony for the hepatitis B program until the fears subsided, so as not to interfere with the educational efforts of the new program.

The report made clear that in order for it to succeed the local population had to be intimately involved in any vaccination project, and it proposed using the tetanus debacle to reinforce the hepatitis program's commitment to work "from the people and towards the people,"[13] an approach that supported the Task Force's basic philosophy.

The Task Force Is Invited into Egypt

Although the Task Force's major commitment on the African continent was in Kenya and Cameroon, it also became involved in two separate Egyptian initiatives. (As part of its growing awareness of the hepatitis B problem in the Middle East, it added a distinguished Jordanian hepatitis expert, Dr. Ala Toukan, to the Task Force.) The first of the Egyptian projects concerned the possibility of transferring recombinant DNA production technology to VACSERA (the Egyptian organization for biological and vaccine production). This rather complex enterprise well illustrates exactly how important a player the Task Force had become in the international arena.

In 1989 Egypt received an unsolicited proposal from Merck to transfer DNA technology for both measles and hepatitis B vaccines. USAID-Cairo, when approached for funding, asked the Task Force and PATH to send a team to evaluate the technical and economic feasibility of the transfer and to determine the feasibility of integrating the hepatitis B vaccine into the Egyptian EPI.[14] (A few months before the team went to Cairo, Maynard himself had been asked by WHO to act as a Temporary WHO Advisor to assess the Egyptian government's interest in a hepatitis B immunization program and the feasibility of local production. This request was in response to the same Merck offer. Again, Maynard was wearing two or three different hats.)[15]

The report issued by the Task Force–PATH team found local production feasible provided that it was combined with the production of other biologicals in an upgraded good manufacturing practices facility. The team also recommended that mass vaccination of infants against hepatitis B be phased into the Egyptian EPI.[16]

However, this Egyptian initiative aggravated a number of latent political conflicts—both inside and outside the Task Force. The external problem resulted from the fact that USAID was sharply divided in its attitude toward the desirability of the technology transfer project. When Maynard made a presentation to the USAID Mission in support of VACSERA's local production it was ill-received. According to a knowledgeable informant, the Economic Section of the Mission "is opposed to all technology transfer that involves the public sector and this reflects an increasingly evident stance on the part of USAID as a whole."[17] Accordingly, the Section did not even suggest specific recommendations for strengthening PATH's feasibility study. Maynard felt that the opposition was clearly political rather than substantive, and the informant agreed that this was the case. The informant found the opposition to Maynard's presentation distasteful, as "witnessed by his statement . . . that the USAID of today is different from the old USAID which he knew to be devoted to the public good."[18] (The anti-transfer position contrasted sharply with the pro-transfer sentiments of USAID workers outside the Economic Section, which had funded the original study and insisted that only VACSERA was a candidate for the Merck technology.)[19]

The Egyptian Intervention Generates Internal Conflicts Within the Task Force

If the internal split within USAID was not bad enough, the Task Force itself was divided on the same issue. As we have seen, Maynard and Mahoney had increasingly opposite views on the feasibility and economic usefulness of local production. Maynard apparently feared that Mahoney's disapproval of the situation in Egypt was so strong that he might unconsciously sabotage the project. Such undermining could occur quite easily, because of the nature of the investigative process and the sensitivity of Egyptian officials. Maynard warned Mahoney,

I think that you might be setting yourself up for a series of criticisms and innuendoes [in the questions you ask] that reflect the very divisive and competitive nature of the cast of characters in the field of gastroenterology and hepatology. In this arena the field is divided into "competitive fiefdoms" of competing individuals who are sure to criticize activities that are not in their own sphere of influence. I feel that you would be entering shark-infested waters . . . that could yield . . . unreliable data about [the extent] of government commitment.[20]

If this type of question were to be reported back to the Ministry of Health, it might be misinterpreted.

As usual, the division within the Task Force was dealt with effectively. Mahoney admitted that as far as he was concerned the Merck project was not the most cost-efficient way for the Egyptian government to get safe, effective, and affordable hepatitis B and measles vaccines. Nevertheless, he supported the proposal because he felt that if USAID was going to spend a lot of money in Egypt, some of it should go to hepatitis B, and certainly Egypt and the Middle East generally would benefit from the development of a modern capacity to manufacture biologics—independent of its cost-effectiveness.[21]

Mahoney, however, was concerned that the Task Force not appear so eager for local production that it would be perceived as not giving adequate weight to other factors. This would perhaps undermine the chances that the Task Force would be invited to advise USAID-Cairo or the Egyptian government in the future. He was also concerned that the Task Force might be seen as a Merck agent because of the two groups' close cooperation on the project. (The danger of having the Task Force's independence questioned never went away.)[22]

The second Egyptian initiative was far less divisive, though also not without conflict. The USAID provided money to vaccinate all babies in the country for hepatitis B. The Task Force was asked to develop health education materials to support that goal. This activity was seen as very important since in Egypt the general population did not even know what hepatitis B was, let alone that their babies needed extra shots. When the Task Force asked the EPI workers in Cairo to include the hepatitis B material in their manuals and educational guides, they refused. So the Task Force went over the workers' heads to the general EPI guide-makers and had it done. As Maynard put it, they "bearded the lion"[23] in Cairo, and the experience was most gratifying.

The Task Force Tries to Open the Soviet Union: A Breakthrough in Uzbekistan

Around the same time the Task Force got involved in the Egyptian venture, it also looked into the possibility of local production in what was then the Soviet Republic of Uzbekistan. Hepatitis B was a major problem in many areas of the Soviet Union; however, the central authorities did not respond adequately to the pressing need for vaccine. Hepatitis B was endemic in Uzbekistan, with carrier rates reaching as high as 17 percent. The Uzbek government became frustrated by Moscow's lack of strategy for vaccine administration or procurement and the absence of any hepatitis B containment policy. The unavailability of vaccine in the Soviet Union and the failure to obtain it through the Ministry of Health in Moscow led the Uzbek government to invite Maynard to visit Tashkent to conduct a preliminary evaluation of the situation.[24]

Maynard was initially anxious about making such an exploratory visit since he knew of the long and fruitless efforts to initiate hepatitis B vaccine production in the Soviet Union. He also knew that currency difficulties could make purchase of vaccine from abroad impossible, and that the central government might not allow Uzbekistan to undertake unilateral initiatives with outsiders. However, Maynard received encouragement to pursue the issue from WHO's Mark Kane and Yuri Ghendon (a Russian national). As conditions evolved in the Soviet Union it became clear that Uzbekistan could indeed make its own independent agreements. When Maynard visited Tashkent he was greeted by the Prime Minister, who informed him that hepatitis B was being given the highest priority. The government was so interested in the possibility of local production that it offered to use some of its limited hard currency reserves to fund a feasibility study through the Task Force. Maynard later met the Secretary of the Communist Party, who said that hepatitis B was a "politically significant issue and that the political will of the Communist Party organs would be placed behind the effort."[25]

Maynard felt that the republic had the infrastructure necessary to produce plasma-derived hepatitis B vaccine, but that for such manufacture to be economical it would have to supply not only itself but the other Asian Soviet republics as well. The Uzbek project was an exciting possibility not only in itself but as a first step in opening up the entire Soviet Union. Maynard hoped that the Task Force could offer the Soviet National Ministry of Health assistance in the creation and implementation of a national program of hepatitis B immunization. If that occurred, the most likely means for providing help would be through WHO, with Task Force members participating in the capacity of WHO Temporary Advisors.[26]

An International Meeting Endorses Universal Hepatitis B Immunization

Task Force activities in different nations continued to expand. Its greatest achievement since the initiation of the Indonesian bid and tender agreement occurred in October 1991 with the convening of an international conference on hepatitis B in Yaounde, Cameroon. The conference was a joint WHO–Task Force venture, and it definitively demonstrated the commanding position the Task Force had achieved in the international arena.[27] The conference brought together 150 participants from more than fifty countries, representatives of international organizations and ministries of health from North and South America, Asia, Africa, Europe, and the Pacific Islands. It included delegates from five of WHO's six regions and representatives from the major vaccine manufacturers, public health experts, and bilateral donors.

A WHO representative announced in the keynote address that universal infant immunization with hepatitis B vaccine was under way in thirty different countries and an additional twenty were ready to begin but lacked the financial resources. The high point of the conference occurred when the participants issued "The Yaounde Declaration on the Elimination of Hepatitis B Infection," which announced that hepatitis B was "comparable to the world's most serious disease and exceeds those of diphtheria, pertussis, polio, cholera, rotavirus diarrhea, and AIDS."[28] It urged that hepatitis B be seen as a children's issue because it kills the parents of young children and is acquired in childhood.[29] Hepatitis B vaccine was the first vaccine against a human cancer, and it could be effectively integrated into the EPI without diminishing that program; thus the conference called on the world and its leaders to recognize the significance of hepatitis B and the rights of children to gain protection from it. Conference participants called for the establishment of a global fund to purchase and deliver the vaccine and for the integration of hepatitis B into the EPI.

The Declaration of Yaounde Is Approved by the EPI and a Timetable Is Adopted

To make the declaration an effective call to action rather than just a symbolic gesture, a number of participants agreed to bring the document to the World Health Assembly (the controlling body for WHO) and work to have it formally adopted. Before that could occur, the declaration was to be read at the 1991 EPI Global Advisory Group (GAG) meeting in Turkey, where it was enthusiastically endorsed. More than that, a timetable for the integration of hepatitis B into the EPI was proposed by the head of the EPI, Robert Kim-Farley, M.D., which meant that the conference's lofty sentiments were being rapidly translated into reality. The GAG called for the integration of hepatitis B immunization into the EPI by 1995 in all countries with hepatitis B carrier rates of 8 percent or greater, and by 1997 in all other countries. (The GAG went on to say that in countries with carrier rates of 2 percent and greater, the best strategy was universal childhood vaccination. Countries with lower rates could consider immunization of adolescents as an addition or alternative to the infant-oriented policy.) The GAG also called for the establishment of a global vaccine fund by 1993 and suggested that the new Children's Vaccine Initiative give high priority to the creation of such a fund.[30]

The remarkable EPI GAG endorsement clearly supported the Task Force's belief that the Yaounde Conference would be seen as a landmark in the history of the fight against hepatitis B. The EPI had supported the adoption of hepatitis B as a universal vaccine at its meetings ever since 1987, but this endorsement constituted a qualitatively different type of support because verbal assurances had been replaced by action.[31]

The EPI's Ambivalent Attitude Toward Hepatitis B Vaccination

The EPI had for years shown a marked ambivalence toward hepatitis B. When the Task Force was in the process of formation, Dr. Ralph Henderson of the EPI had offered interest and encouragement[32] that had been vital at such a crucial stage of development. He had made it clear, however, that existing hepatitis B vaccine prices made it impossible for the EPI to be involved with the disease, and he doubted that the Task Force could change the situation in the near future. Henderson's personal philosophy for the EPI, of which he was the driving creative force, was opposed to taking hasty actions on any issue. As late as July 1990 Henderson said:

The *long term goal*[33] is the integration [of hepatitis B] into EPI. . . . [But] cost determines how enthusiastic we can be in pushing the policy. As price goes down, the debate heats up. . . . [However,] resources are still low, it is a new demand on health resources. . . . One can be frustrated by the slowness of the official process but in hepatitis B I want to see a constituency build up, rather than going too fast and losing some support. It looks like [I am] not being enough of an advocate . . . [but] EPI has tried to do things well [and I feel] gradual development is best.[34]

Henderson felt there were many practical problems that had to be dealt with before any aggressive action could be taken. For example, in Africa it was important not to get financial donors excited and then disappointed by the poor performance of countries that did not administer vaccines well. In addition, one had to know the different doses of vaccine and the best times to administer it—all of which would take time. Sensitivity to local problems—such as the inability of many countries to administer hepatitis vaccination at birth—was also important. Thus, according to Henderson, only a general recommendation, not a specific one, made sense at this time.[35]

Moderate and gradual change was not the Task Force's goal, nor was moving slowly while infinite numbers of practical questions were definitively answered. Rather, the Task Force members felt that this approach, which was dominant at WHO as well as at the EPI, had kept hepatitis B a back-burner issue and would continue to do so for decades to come.

Henderson saw himself as an advocate for hepatitis B, and he felt he had helped shape the EPI so that it worked as an institutionalized supporter for new vaccines. But according to Dr. Kenneth Warren, who worked with Henderson on the Task Force for Child Survival, Henderson's innate conservatism and methodicalness made the EPI "move so slowly . . . [because] . . . everything new he gets hit with, he says 'no' at first, then he adjusts."[36] This left him ill-equipped to be the type of product champion that Henderson himself contended a new vaccine required.[37] Many of the EPI regional representatives, especially in Africa, were also prone to knee-jerk negative responses to anyone "prematurely" agitating for the hepatitis B issue.

A New Head for the EPI Means a More Aggressive Policy on Fighting Hepatitis B

Nevertheless, in a sea of hostility and indifference, Henderson and his EPI constituted one of the more open-minded and relatively friendly forces. Henderson may not have taken the lead on hepatitis B, but he offered little active opposition and a fair amount of moderate support.[38]

Later, the situation improved markedly under the new head of the EPI, Dr. Robert Kim-Farley. Kim-Farley was a guest at a Task Force Interim Meeting in Geneva in June 1991, a few months before the Yaounde Conference. Alfred Prince said that the purpose of the meeting was to discuss the lack of real progress in integrating hepatitis B vaccine into the EPI. Kim-Farley wanted to know what the Task Force could do to accelerate progress. He felt that the new Children's Vaccine Initiative (an organization created by the Rockefeller Foundation, WHO, UNICEF, the United Nations Development Programme, and the World Bank) should have hepatitis B as its lead project, and, indeed, he believed the key to the introduction of other new vaccines into the EPI would depend on the success of the hepatitis B vaccine. When asked how to get the hepatitis vaccine as the official seventh EPI antigen, he said the EPI would be placed on the 1992 World Health Assembly agenda, and it might be possible to bring forward the Cairo GAG recommendation on hepatitis B and get official endorsement. Kim-Farley recommended that the Task Force

continue to argue that HBV [hepatitis B vaccine] is a universal immunogen, that the Task Force be prepared to make some small statement to the W[orld] H[ealth] A[ssembly of WHO], convince UNICEF to classify HBV as a Noted Project which allows donors to earmark funds for that purpose, and to lobby [the] C[hildren's] V[accine] I[nitiative] to include HBV in its priorities.[39]

If Kim-Farley's words at the Task Force meeting sounded supportive, his actions in October 1991, at the EPI GAG held in Turkey, proved he was an ally: he called for a hepatitis B timetable to actualize the EPI's commitment to universal vaccination. Kim-Farley held that it made no sense to develop new vaccines when existing vaccines, such as hepatitis B, were not being brought into the EPI.[40]

Support and Opposition for Hepatitis B Vaccination at the EPI Conference in Turkey

The victory in Turkey, however, was not complete. Significant conflict flared up at the meeting and highlighted how far the Task Force still remained from total success. The adoption of the timetable for hepatitis B was fiercely opposed by Terrell Hill, the Advisor to the EPI for UNICEF.[41] While Hill was not able to win over the majority of delegates to his view, the success of the GAG's recommendations ultimately depended upon UNICEF's attitude, which he represented.

The reason for UNICEF's pivotal significance was that the EPI did not provide funding for the six universal vaccines. Rather, most of the money was supplied by UNICEF, and it saw the growing momentum of the hepatitis B campaign as a major threat to its solvency and its freedom to make decisions. In Hill's eyes the problem for UNICEF was quite simple:

We would love everyone to be immunized against hepatitis B. The problem we have had for the last eight to nine years is we have been seen as the court of last resort to provide vaccine to the developing world. As a gift!!!. . . . [And] EPI/WHO and the Task Force hope that we will pay for the vaccine.[42]

Hill went on to say that Kane of WHO had estimated that the cost of the hepatitis B program would be approximately $120 million, but he did not say who would pay for it. At the same time the EPI was pushing hepatitis B, it was calling for the complete eradication of polio and had moved the timetable for that goal from the year 2000 down to 1995. The price tag for that campaign was $79 million. Although Rotary International had purchased most of the polio vaccine, it intended to phase down its contribution and would run out of money before the job was completed. UNICEF would be expected to pick up the shortfall. In addition, Hill continued,

[W]e have a measles goal: control by 1995. There will be a doubling of our investment on measles. Also there is a neo-natal tetanus goal; [that] will [require] double the investment. The bottom line is we don't have the resources. . . . We have other goals [too]—education, jobs, etc. All require more funds. If we fundraise where do we put the emphasis. . . . [If UNICEF started to raise funds aggressively for hepatitis B, then] that money will not be available for AIDS, diarrheal disease . . . or education. . . . [It is a case of] competition with scarce resources.[43]

As far as UNICEF was concerned, hepatitis B, despite the tremendous price drop brought about by the Task Force, was still a very expensive vaccine. The other six EPI vaccines as a group cost only about $.65 per child. Hepatitis B, at $1 a dose, would raise the price to immunize each child to $3.65![44] While Kane claimed that hepatitis B vaccine could be obtained at $.50 a dose (and the Task Force believed it could ultimately go as low as $.10–$.15 in massive orders), Hill was highly skeptical, saying it was too easy to speculate about cheap prices.

Hill also felt that substantial technical problems concerning hepatitis B vaccine continued to exist which its proponents had ignored but which UNICEF could not; for example, whether they should use plasma-derived vaccine or recombinant DNA. If they went ahead with the single hepatitis B vaccine and a multivalent combination vaccine came out, a new financial problem would develop. A host of questions existed about dosage levels, the interchangeability of DNA and plasma vaccines, and other technical matters that made it foolish to rush ahead before these questions were resolved. UNICEF would not buy any vaccine without WHO's Biologicals division's approval—and this had not been given for hepatitis B.

The list of UNICEF objections to moving quickly on hepatitis B seemed endless, and the items all seemed very reasonable and insurmountable, at least for many years to come. But if the Task Force had accepted such hard-headed realism, mass hepatitis B immunization would never have become a real possibility.

(It is good to remember that UNICEF's coolness to the hepatitis B issue goes back all the way to the formation of the International Task Force. When Mahoney was invited by Kenneth Warren to address the Task Force for Child Survival, the greatest opposition to his presentation came from Newton Bowles, the UNICEF representative. Bowles's position—which in Warren's view reflected that of James Grant, the head of UNICEF—was that hepatitis B was not a childhood disease problem because it did not directly kill children. Maynard, Mahoney, and Prince spent years trying to convince donors and international agencies that a non-lethal infection acquired in childhood that later led to their deaths when they were parents was indeed a killer of children. They had a great deal of success, even at UNICEF, but it was far from total.)

The EPI GAG that met in Turkey was seen as a major threat to UNICEF. It replaced the earlier and more comfortably vague Cairo GAG recommendation with an unpalatable timetable. The only bright spot for UNICEF was that the timetable was slower than that recommended by the Declaration of Yaounde. The GAG called for integration of hepatitis B into the EPI by 1995 only in countries having a carrier incidence of 8 percent or higher, while Yaounde did not contain a minimum carrier rate qualification. (Indeed, there were many at the GAG meeting who wanted the faster timetable.)[45]

Hill was dismayed by the rapidity with which the hepatitis B resolutions were passed. The discussion lasted only one hour and came at the end of a long meeting. Kane, fresh from the Cameroon Conference, made a powerful presentation and, despite the absence of hepatitis B experts at the GAG meeting, won over the non-hepatitis specialists.[46] The main opposition, other than that of the UNICEF spokesman, came from Northern European countries with low hepatitis rates. The most outspoken opponent of universal vaccination was David Salisbury, M.D., of Great Britain, who was appalled by the idea of spending money for a minor disease when other, more pressing ones went begging. He felt the recommendation for hepatitis vaccination should only apply to countries with high carrier rates.[47] While Hill found a number of supporters for his position, they did not carry the meeting. However, Hill noticed that none of the major donor groups present at the GAG spoke out for hepatitis B (or polio eradication for that matter). As he put it, "The donors weren't falling over themselves to fund this."[48]

Fortunately, while UNICEF was opposed to taking on the financial burden of hepatitis B immunization, it was not opposed to lending its services to countries that could raise their own funds to establish national programs. UNICEF was willing to help create a consortium mechanism by which countries could pool their individual requirements and have UNICEF purchase the vaccine from the manufacturers at substantial savings. This type of aid was quite substantial and not very costly to UNICEF. The problem that the EPI GAG created was that it gave hepatitis B equal priority with measles, tetanus, and polio control. Also, according to Hill, "If . . . implemented by WHO I will have 100 UNICEF offices pressured by their countries to [directly] buy hepatitis B—that is the real life situation!"[49] No one would settle for a self-funded consortium once WHO declared hepatitis B the seventh universal vaccine.

The Task Force's Response to UNICEF's Objections

Clearly, with UNICEF having so many reservations about hepatitis B, the Task Force still had a major job left to do. Its Yaounde Declaration and EPI recommendations were landmark achievements, but without a funding source universal hepatitis B vaccination would not be achievable. Nevertheless, the situation looked favorable. Hill's fears of being stampeded on the hepatitis B issue reflected the political reality that

UNICEF could be pressured into moving by growing international concern. The Task Force continued to step up its contacts with Ministers of Health, bilateral donors, manufacturers, and other opinion makers as a means of keeping the hepatitis momentum going.

In dealing with UNICEF the Task Force was also aided by its increasingly close ties with both the EPI and WHO. After Kim-Farley became head of the EPI he told Task Force members he needed their assistance to "jaw-bone" both UNICEF and individual donors[50] and asked them to lobby the World Health Assembly on the hepatitis issue[51] (since the EPI was forbidden to exert pressure on it). In addition, the close working ties forged by WHO and the Task Force in co-sponsoring the Yaounde Conference were to some extent institutionalized when the Task Force asked Kane to formally become a member of the group.[52] When WHO gave Kane the permission to join, it provided a public link to the long-standing personal bonds among Kane, Maynard, and the Task Force. All of these activities and connections could be mobilized to put pressure on UNICEF.[53] Today, nevertheless, the Task Force remains aware that their best policy is to win over the UNICEF staff by persuasion and diplomacy. With all of UNICEF's reluctance and anxiety, it is nevertheless dedicated to the fight against disease; it has a mandate to lower child mortality; and it is aware that hepatitis B has an impact on childhood mortality because it kills parents.[54] UNICEF workers like to see themselves as bold pioneers, and in the long run they can be convinced to be supportive.[55]

The Task Force, while totally opposed to UNICEF's go-slow position, was not oblivious to the many problems Hill spoke about. It knew that the price UNICEF pays for all its vaccines was going up rapidly and that UNICEF was justifiably feeling besieged. (Or as Maynard put it, "The European drug companies are doing the typical capitalistic tactic—withholding supplies to drive up the price.")[56] However, the Task Force's position was that the obstacles, whether financial or technical, were challenges that must be actively met and mastered, not reasons for delay. For example, the development of a combined diphtheria-pertussis-tetanus-hepatitis B vaccine was a major goal of the Task Force, which continues to encourage manufacturers to produce one and to solve dosage and schedule problems. However, the Task Force saw no reason to delay the beginning of a national program until the new vaccine was ready for the market. The extra costs and inconvenience of switching vaccines may be real, but they are minor compared with getting the program off the ground. Each year's delay means countless deaths from cirrhosis and liver cancer in thirty or forty years. It is that haunting awareness of mortality, not zealotry or a lack of concern for or understanding of practical problems, that drove the aggressiveness of the Task Force, which has always combined its acute concern about neutralizing practical restraints with its dedication to forceful and rapid action. The criticism that the Task Force is overly idealistic is simply not convincing.

Conclusion

While the war against hepatitis B and liver cancer has not yet been finally won, the fight is now well advanced. The new WHO guidelines, combined with universal vaccination programs even in such countries as the United States, raise the real possibility that hepatitis B will ultimately go the way of smallpox—to total eradication.[57] The disease has no animal reservoir, and when it ceases to be passed from human to human it will be eradicated. The end of the hepatitis B pandemic will in turn eliminate 80 percent of the primary liver cancer in the world, paradoxically making infectious disease researchers, rather than cancer scientists, the most successful warriors in the war against cancer. (It is widely believed among those working with hepatitis B that if the vaccine had been developed by cancer researchers rather than infectious disease scientists and heralded as the first, and only, anti-cancer vaccine, there would have been no long delays in funding of the vaccination programs or the extended period of non-benign neglect that the vaccine experienced.) The possibility of eradication owes much to the practical idealism of a small group of woolly-headed, quixotic scientists and public servants called the International Task Force on Hepatitis B Immunization.

Whether hepatitis B is totally eliminated from humankind in the future or not, the Task Force's present accomplishments stand as a model for enlightened and determined social activism. The Task Force was successful in achieving its four established goals; first, to force down the unconscionable price of the vaccine; second, to make hepatitis B (and its associated liver cancer) a top priority issue for both the leaders of the chief international health organizations and the nations of the developing world; third, to interest the large pharmaceutical companies in the mass hepatitis B immunization market and to abandon their concentration on the high-profit/small-demand middle- and upper-class population; and fourth, to prove that developing countries, even under adverse conditions, could successfully carry out hepatitis vaccination programs and integrate them into the EPI.

To achieve these goals the Task Force had to convince the international arbiters of health that hepatitis B was a legitimate part of the war against childhood diseases, that its indirect death rate (from cancer and cirrhosis) rivaled or surpassed that of measles. It had to encourage the pharmaceutical concerns to compete for developing world business, but not in a way that destroyed their weaker competitors or undermined public confidence in the vaccines. It had to help change the international biological standards that artificially prevented safe and effective vaccines from meeting WHO standards, which had made Third World governments reluctant to use the cheapest products. To succeed it had to deal sensitively with the cultures and politics of Thailand, Indonesia, Kenya, and Cameroon, and it had to deal skillfully with the personal, bureaucratic, and turf wars that characterize the health politics of WHO, UNICEF, and other international organizations. At the same time, in order to maintain its effectiveness and unity as an organization, the Task Force had to successfully weather its own internal conflicts and disagreements: PATH versus the Task Force, the ideological disputes over public versus private sector competency, disagreements over the desirability of technology transfer, the claims of egoism among a group of strong-willed men and women, the desire to put personal or group ambition, pride, and fame above cooperation and goal achievement. The Task Force did all these things.

How were these goals accomplished? Who could have predicted that any of these achievements would come to pass? Some answers are fairly clear. First, success was possible because of a window of opportunity created by the rise of the Pacific Rim countries that were eager and willing to break into the world market. In the case of hepatitis B the Korean pharmaceutical companies and such giant financial powerhouses as the Samsung conglomerate were vital resources. Hungry entrepreneurs meant that competition in the vaccine field was a real possibility. Alfred Prince, with his simplified, less costly hepatitis vaccine technology and his technology transfer to Samsung's Cheil Sugar Company, was a major force in opening that window of opportunity.

Richard Mahoney and PATH also were indispensable for the formation and success of the Task Force. Mahoney was the catalyst for the creation of the group. Without him it would not have come into existence. The other members of the Task Force would have continued to champion the hepatitis issue but in a much less effective way. Unity was their strength, and Mahoney's combination of idealism and pragmatism, of social dedication and personal ambition, of man-on-the-move entrepreneur and altruist, was a potent and irrepressible force. Supporting Mahoney was PATH—an organization that shared many of his characteristics. Without PATH as its secretariat, the Task Force would have failed. A small group of dedicated part-time reformers could not have accomplished what they set out to do. They needed the staff expertise and resources that only PATH could provide, as well as PATH's knowledge of and contacts with potential funding sources.

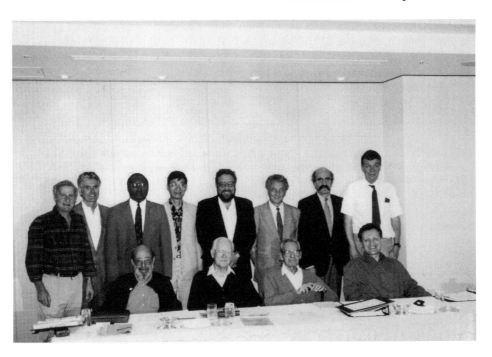

Tokyo Task Force meeting, May 1993. *Left to right, back row:* Dr. Ian Gust, Dr. Richard Mahoney, Dr. Clement Kiire, Dr. Xu Xi-Yi, Dr. Mark Kane, Dr. Yuri Ghendon, Dr. Oscar Fay, Dr. James Maynard; *front row:* Dr. Alfred Prince, Dr. Joseph Melnick, Dr. Saul Krugman, Dr. Alain Goudeau.

Many members of the Task Force wanted to believe that PATH was simply an instrument that could be used or discarded at will, since they feared being dominated by their service organization. The reality was different: PATH was indispensable.

But Mahoney and PATH could not have effectively functioned by themselves. They lacked the expertise and the prestige that the scientists of the Task Force possessed. PATH's staff lacked the credentials of James Maynard, Alfred Prince, R. Palmer Beasley, Ian Gust, or Alain Goudeau. There were doors in Asia, Africa, Washington, and Geneva that would not open to Mahoney or to PATH, but only to scientists with international reputations.

Of the many prominent people on the Task Force none was more vital than Maynard, who was essential to the successful functioning of the group. The choice of Maynard as a Vice President of PATH had been inspired. Maynard, as head of the Hepatitis Branch of the Centers for Disease Control, was a man accustomed to exercising authority and dealing with those at the highest levels of the health world. While he was a leading American public health official, he was deeply concerned with the international arena. He was ironed-willed, with deep ideological and philosophical commitments to the public good; equally important, he loved a good fight. He got extreme pleasure when he could announce that the Task Force was successfully "bearding the lion"— whether it was WHO, of which he was a major advisor, or an obstructive American governmental agency. Nothing could bring a smile to his face as quickly as talk about how "the shit was going to hit the fan" as the Task Force pushed and prodded one slow-moving bureaucracy after another. He was neither a man of faint heart nor one who suffered fools gladly. His name alone, and certainly his actual appearance in a country, could convince a Minister of Health that a vaccine was acceptable or a program practical. His dual role as Task Force member and WHO Advisor made it possible to win over or counter key officials in WHO— necessary feats if the Task Force was to achieve its goals. Without Maynard, success would not have been possible.

Could a group of concerned scientists like those who made up the Task Force succeed in other health areas? I believe it could, but it would require a similar mix. The group would have to be composed of scientists of the highest reputation. At least some of them would have to combine idealism with political savvy and aggressive confidence. The group would have to enlist the services of an organization such as PATH, since the former could not function without the latter. If it could then tolerate differences of opinion and subordinate individual egoism to its stated goal, it would have a chance of bringing about effective public policy. Individuals like Mahoney, Maynard, and Prince were indispensable in the fight against hepatitis B, but they are not unique in the world of science.

Update

When the World Health Assembly finally met in May 1992, it endorsed the goal of universal hepatitis B immunization by the year 1997. There were many who thus believed that the usefulness of the Task Force had finally come to an end. Even John Bruer of the McDonnell Foundation raised the question of the future purpose of the group. Representatives of WHO, however, insisted that the Task Force still had a critical role to play. The growing crisis in funding for other universal vaccines— created by the combination of cost increases and donor fatigue— continues to make finding money for hepatitis B implementation problematic. Though a hepatitis shot is now only $0.55 a dose, it is nevertheless comparatively expensive.[58] In addition, new diseases are competing for the limited available resources (e.g., the hemophilias B and pneumococcal vaccines).

The Task Force now has to push for what Maynard calls new quantum leaps to protect its success. It believes the cost of the vaccine can still be reduced significantly, perhaps to as low as $0.15 a dose. The Task Force is also stepping up its efforts to encourage manufacturers to combine hepatitis B with other vaccines—especially diphtheria-pertussis-tetanus—both to lower the cost and to link it physically to established vaccines whose funding cannot be cut off. Task Force members are currently in the process of looking at the dozens of Asian pharmaceutical companies that produce diphtheria-pertussis-tetanus vaccines, with the goal of helping the best of them (including Indonesia's BioFarma and the Thai Government Pharmaceutical Organization) to upgrade their product, achieve good manufacturing standards, and successfully combine hepatitis B with the other three vaccines. Clearly, for the Task Force the challenge continues.[59]

As of October 1994, seventy-three nations had begun to establish, or had announced their intentions to establish, national hepatitis B vaccination programs. They represent half the countries of the world and include 40 percent of the world's children and 60 percent of the global carriers of the hepatitis B virus.[60] In addition, UNICEF, in a major change of policy, declared that it would provide funds for the purchase of hepatitis B vaccine to all poor countries that requested funding and whose carrier rates were 5 percent or greater (contingent upon the availability of funds).[61]

Notes

1. "A Model Hepatitis B Immunization Programme in the Republic of Cameroon (Draft Protocol)," by the Ministry of Health, Ministry of Higher Education and Research, Republic of Cameroon, Task Force, Program for Appropriate Technology in Health, and WHO, June 1989.

2. Memo by Richard Mahoney to James Maynard, May 23, 1988.

3. Memo by Richard Mahoney to James Maynard, June 7, 1988, assessing the conditions in Kenya.

4. "A Model Program for Hepatitis B Immunization in EMBU District, Kenya," draft protocol by the Ministry of Health, Government of Kenya, Task Force, and Program for Appropriate Technology in Health, May 1989.

5. Memo by Mahoney to James Maynard, June 7, 1988, concerning the assessment in Kenya.

6. Memo by Viven Tsu to Dr. Clement Kiire, April 11, 1989.

7. Ibid.

8. "A Model Program for Hepatitis B Immunization in EMBU District, Kenya," draft protocol by the Ministry of Health, Government of Kenya, Task Force, and PATH, May 1989.

9. Interview with Maynard, June 25, 1991.

10. "1991 Annual Narrative and Interim Financial Report to the James S. McDonnell Foundation," from the International Task Force on Hepatitis B Immunization, submitted by PATH, December 1991.

11. Ibid.

12. "Hepatitis B Vaccination Project, Anti-Tetanus Toxoid (ATT) Vaccination and the Rumour of Sterilization in the North West Province, Cameroon: Anatomy of a Boomerang," by Emmanuel Yenshu (this report is attached to "Model Hepatitis B Vaccination Project," Second Progress Report, the Centre Universitaire Des Sciences De La Santa, Yaounde, Peter Ndumbe, M.D., Ph.D., Project Director, covering July 1–October 1, 1990.

13. Ibid.

14. "1990 Annual Narrative and Financial Report to The James S. McDonnell Foundation" from the International Task Force on Hepatitis B Immunization, March 1991.

15. "Consultant Report: James Maynard, WHO Temporary Advisor, WHO Regional Office for the Middle East, Alexandria Egypt, December 3–7, 1989."

16. Ibid.

17. Memo by Maynard to Mahoney concerning a telephone conversation with Jim Sarn, June 6, 1990.

18. Ibid.

19. Ibid.

20. Memo by Maynard to Mahoney, February 27, 1990.

21. Memo by Mahoney to Maynard, August 31, 1990.

22. Ibid.

23. Interview with Maynard, October 25, 1991.

24. Memo by Maynard, August 3, 1990.

25. Memo by Maynard to Task Force members concerning the trip to the Soviet Union, May 30, 1990.

26. Ibid.

27. The Task Force worked closely with Kane on the conference. Relations with him were friendly. However, because Kane was an official of WHO, one had to be diplomatic to avoid institutional conflict. Mahoney told Kane that he and the Task Force wanted to have a key role in drafting the WHO guidelines on the integration of hepatitis B vaccine into the EPI and offered to write a first draft. Kane was enthusiastic and asked if Mahoney could come to Geneva for a few weeks. However, Kane needed to get approval from his superiors. Mahoney informed Maynard: "I believe that while Mark is willing to give the Task Force a prominent role in drafting the document, he wants to assure that it is seen as a 'WHO' document and not a Task Force document that WHO has adopted." Mahoney thought that a very reasonable "and probably unswayable view" (Mahoney to Maynard, October 25, 1990).

28. "The Yaounde Declaration on the Elimination of Hepatitis B Infection," issued by the International Conference on the Control of Hepatitis B in the Developing World, October 1991.

29. It was Mahoney's hope that some time in "the next ten years we wouldn't have to say hepatitis B helps kids by saving parents—we can say it [the vaccine] is useful by itself" (interview with Mahoney, April 29, 1991).

30. See "Expanded Programme on Immunization," reprinted from *WHO Weekly Epidemiological Record*, No. 3, pp. 11–15; No. 4, pp. 17–19; No. 5, pp. 27–30, 1992. The fund would be for new vaccines in general, not just hepatitis B.

31. Interview with Maynard, October 25, 1991.

32. Maynard went to the Washington Immunization Conference in 1986 and presented a cost-benefit analysis (written by Kane) that showed that a hepatitis B immunization program was comparable in cost-effectiveness to live measles vaccination. Henderson asked Maynard to submit an official letter to the EPI requesting that a working group be convened to consider adding hepatitis B to the list of immunizable disease (memo by Mahoney to Hepatitis B File, July 9, 1986).

33. Emphasis added.

34. Interview with Henderson, July 19, 1990.

35. Ibid.

36. Interview with Kenneth Warren, November 18, 1991.

37. Interview with Henderson, July 19, 1990.

38. In an interview, John Clements, M.D., of the EPI, spoke as if Henderson and the EPI were the driving force behind the movement to large-scale hepatitis B vaccination. Henderson, in a later interview, took a more modest position but one that was basically supportive of Clements's claim. The evidence does not support this position.

39. "Interim Meeting of the International Task Force on Hepatitis B Immunization," Geneva, June 11–12, 1991.

40. Interview with Terrell Hill, Advisor to the EPI for UNICEF, November 11, 1991.

41. Hill's vehement opposition came as a surprise to Task Force members because he had been seen for years as the major supporter of hepatitis B at UNICEF (interview with Maynard, October 21, 1991).

42. Interview with Hill, November 11, 1991.

43. Ibid.

44. Comment by Kane at the "Interim Meeting of the International Task Force," Geneva, June 11–12, 1991.

45. Interview with Hill, November 11, 1991.

46. Ibid.

47. Ibid. Kane told the Task Force (at the interim meeting in Geneva) that a European Regional Office of WHO working group had recommended that all European children receive hepatitis B vaccine. This had received support from southern and eastern European countries, many of which have very high carrier rates. It was less well received by European countries in other parts of the continent.

48. Ibid.

49. Ibid.

50. Interview with Maynard, June 18, 1991.

51. "Interim Meeting of the International Task Force," Geneva, June 11–12, 1991.

52. In addition to asking Kane to join, they asked Drs. Saul Krugman and Joseph Melnick, two towering figures in the field of infectious disease research, to be special advisors to the Task Force (memo by Maynard to Task Force members, March 4, 1992).

53. The people at UNICEF are also not ignorant of the effects of hepatitis B.

Hill told me that one of his colleagues and friends had died of liver cancer related to hepatitis B. Such direct knowledge helps shape attitudes.

54. Interview with Hill, November 11, 1991.

55. In fact, some Task Force members did not see a major problem with UNICEF at all. As Mahoney put it: "Don't presume that UNICEF has not been cooperative. I think that is a bum rap. It is a procurement agency. They don't have the money, yet. People are shooting the messenger. They don't have enough donor money to buy EPI vaccines—let alone a new vaccine. . . . UNICEF is pro-HB [hepatitis B]. But [there is] still not enough money." According to Mahoney the problem was not UNICEF's attitude but the fact that WHO and UNICEF were engaged in a "turf war" over their respective roles in the fight for world health. According to Mahoney, when James Grant became head of UNICEF he championed the concept of GOBI (growth monitoring, oral rehydration, breast feeding, immunization) as the goal of the organization. All of these processes, with the exception of literacy, are health interventions, which traditionally come under the mandate of WHO. WHO has felt that its prerogatives were being taken away. The new Children's Vaccine Initiative, according to Mahoney, is also part of the competition between the two organizations. In his view it is vital that the Task Force not be drawn into the dispute and forced to take sides (interview with Mahoney, June 20, 1991). This obviously is a real problem given the Task Force's increasingly strong links to the EPI and WHO. (For more information on the UNICEF-WHO fight see June Goodfield, *A Chance to Live: The Heroic Story of the Global Campaign to Immunize the World's Children* [New York: Macmillan, 1991], passim.)

56. Interview with Maynard, October 25, 1991.

57. See Baruch Blumberg, "Hepatitis B Virus and the Carrier Problem," in *In Time of Plague* (Special Issue), *Social Research* 55(3) (1988): 405, where he presents eradication of hepatitis B as a possibility. The issue of whether diseases other than smallpox can be totally eliminated is debated by a number of experts in *World Health Forum* 2(2) (1981): 281–90.

58. Because UNICEF feels that buying hepatitis B vaccine will take resources from other programs it "has set an arbitrary target of $0.25/dose before it begins to buy the vaccine for donation to national immunization programs"; thus $0.55 is still much too high (Anthony Robbins and Phyllis Freeman, "International Childhood Vaccine Initiative," *Pediatric Infectious Disease Journal* 12 [1993]: 523–27).

59. Interview with Maynard, July 7, 1993.

60. Mark Kane, speaking to the Scientific Advisory Group of Experts (SAGE) meeting, Global Programme for Vaccines and Immunization, World Health Organization, Geneva, October 17–19, 1994.

61. "Sustaining Immunization and Assuring Vaccines for the World's Children: A Strategy for UNICEF," Executive Director's policy directive, prepared by Amie Bateson, Terrel M. Hill, and David J. Halliday, October 5, 1994 (unpublished), distributed at the SAGE meeting of the Global Programme for Vaccines and Immunization, World Health Organization, Geneva, October 17–19, 1994. As of November 3, 1994, the authorization to create the new policy at UNICEF had been obtained, but James Grant had yet to formally sign the document. Despite continued internal opposition to the policy change, the signing was expected to take place by the end of the year.

Selected Bibliography

Banerji, Debabar. "Crash of the Immunization Program: Consequences of a Totalitarian Approach." *International Journal of Health Services* 20 (1990): 501–10.

———. "Hidden Menace in the Universal Child Immunization Program." *International Journal of Health Services* 18 (1988): 293–99.

Benenson, Abram S., ed. *Control of Communicable Diseases in Man.* Washington, D.C.: American Public Health Association, 1985.

Blumberg, Baruch. "Hepatitis B Virus and the Carrier Problem." *Social Research* 55 (Autumn 1988): 401–12.

Blumberg, B. S., B. J. S. Gerstley, D. A. Hungerford, W. T. London, and A. I. Sutnick. "A Serum Antigen (Australia Antigen) in Down's Syndrome, Leukemia and Hepatitis." *Annals of Internal Medicine* 66 (1967): 924–31.

Blumberg, B. S., W. T. London, A. I. Sutnick, F. R. Camp, Jr., A. J. Luzzio, and N. F. Conte. "Hepatitis Carriers Among Soldiers Who Have Returned from Vietnam: Australia Antigen Studies." *Transfusion* 14 (1974): 63–66.

Chetley, Andrew. *Healthy Business? World Health and the Pharmaceutical Industry.* London: Zed Books, 1990.

Girling, John. *Thailand Society and Politics.* Ithaca, N.Y.: Cornell University Press, 1981.

Goodfield, June. *A Chance to Live: The Heroic Story of the Global Campaign to Immunize the World's Children.* New York: Macmillan, 1991.

Gust, Ian. "Control of Hepatitis B in the Western Pacific Region." *Medical Journal of Australia* 144 (1986): 473–74.

———. "Public Health Control of HBV: Worldwide HBV Vaccination Programme." In *The Hepatitis Delta Virus*, edited by John L. Gerin, Robert H. Purcell, and Mario Rizzetto, 333–42. New York: Wiley-Liss, 1991.

———. "Toward the Control of Hepatitis B: An Historical Review." *Australian Paediatric Journal* 22 (1986): 273–76.

Hardy, Anne. *The Epidemic Streets: Infectious Disease and the Rise of Preventive Medicine, 1856–1900.* Oxford: Clarendon Press, 1993.

Hopkins, Jack W. *The Eradication of Smallpox: Organizational Learning and Innovation in International Health.* Boulder, Colo.: Westview Press, 1989.

Jackson, Karl, and Lucian Pye, eds. *Political Power and Communications in Indonesia.* Berkeley, Calif.: University of California Press, 1980.

Kingdon, John W. *Agendas, Alternatives and Public Policies.* New York: HarperCollins Publishers, 1984.

Kiple, Kenneth, ed. *The Cambridge World History of Human Disease*. Cambridge: Cambridge University Press, 1993.

Lam, S. K., C. L. Lai, and E. K. Yeah, eds. *Viral Hepatitis B Infection in the Western Pacific Region: Vaccine and Control*. Hong Kong: World Scientific, 1984.

Lively, Robert. "The American System." *Business History Review* 29 (1955): 81–94.

McKeown, Thomas. *The Role of Medicine: Dream, Mirage, or Nemesis?* Princeton, N.J.: Princeton University Press, 1979.

Muraskin, William. "Hepatitis B as a Model (and Anti-Model) for AIDS." In *AIDS and Contemporary History*, edited by Virginia Berridge and Philip Strong, 108–32. New York: Cambridge University Press, 1993.

———. "Individual Rights Versus the Public Health: The Controversy over the Integration of Retarded Hepatitis B Carriers into the New York City Public School System." *Journal of the History of Medicine and Allied Sciences* 45 (1990): 64–98.

———. "Individual Rights Versus the Public Health: The Problem of the Asian Hepatitis B Carriers in America." *Social Science and Medicine* 36 (1993): 203–16.

———. "The Silent Epidemic: The Social, Ethical, and Medical Problems Surrounding the Fight Against Hepatitis B." *Journal of Social History* 22 (1988): 277–98.

Navarro, Vicente. "A Critique of the Ideological and Political Position of the Brandt Report and the Alma Ata Declaration." *International Journal of Health Services* 14 (1984): 159–73.

Newell, Kenneth. "Selective Primary Health Care: The Counter Revolution." *Social Science and Medicine* 26 (1988): 903–6.

Prince, Alfred. "Prevalence of Serum-Hepatitis-Related Antigen (SH) in Different Geographical Regions." *American Journal of Tropical Medicine and Hygiene* 19 (1970): 872–79.

Prince, A. M. "Detection of Serum Hepatitis Virus Carriers by Testing for the SH (Australia) Antigen: A Review of Current Methodology." *Vox Sanguinus* 9 (1970): 417–24.

Pye, Lucien W. *Asian Power and Politics: The Cultural Dimensions of Authority*. Cambridge, Mass.: Harvard University Press, 1985.

Robbins, Anthony, and Phyllis Freeman. "Obstacles to Developing Vaccines for the Third World." *Scientific American* (November 1988): 90–95.

Szreter, Simon. "The Importance of Social Intervention in Britain's Mortality Decline, c. 1850–1914: A Reinterpretation of the Role of Public Health." *Social History* 1 (1988): 1–37.

Warren, Kenneth S. "The Alma-Ata Declaration: Health for All by the Year 2000?" In *Encyclopedia Britannica, 1990 Year Book*, 21–30. Chicago: Encyclopedia Britannica Inc., 1990.

Warren, Kenneth and Julia Walsh. "Selective Primary Health Care: An Interim Strategy for Disease Control in Developing Countries." *New England Journal of Medicine* 301 (1979): 967–74.

Weisse, Allen B. *Medical Odysseys*. New Brunswick, N.J.: Rutgers University Press, 1991.

WHO Expert Committee on Biological Standardization, *Thirty-first Report, World Health Organization Technical Report Series, No. 658*. Geneva: WHO, 1981.

Wiener, Benjamin. "GOBI versus PHC? Some Dangers of Selective Primary Health Care." *Social Science and Medicine* 26 (1988): 963–69.

Wilson, Leonard. "The Historical Decline of Tuberculosis in Europe and America: Its Causes and Significance." *Journal of History of Medicine and Allied Sciences* 45 (1990): 366–96.

———. "The Rise and Fall of Tuberculosis in Minnesota: The Role of Infection." *Bulletin of the History of Medicine* 66 (1992): 16–52.

Index